THROUGH THE DARKNESS

ONE MAN'S FIGHT TO OVERCOME EPILEPSY

MIKE HENLE

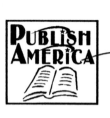

PublishAmerica
Baltimore

First printing

ISBN: 1-4137-7163-7
PUBLISHED BY PUBLISHAMERICA, LLLP
www.publishamerica.com
Baltimore

Printed in the United States of America

This book is dedicated to:

The staff of Scripps Clinic and Scripps Green Hospital for taking the time to turn my life around. In particular, Dr. Andy Aung, Dr. Thomas Waltz, and my clinician Kate Culliton will forever stand out in my life for their efforts.

My family and friends who stuck by me during some very challenging times both before and after my surgery. They were there to pick me up when I fell.

Rudy Ruettiger, whose very timely pep talk gave me the strength to keep going during the writing of the manuscript.

Stephanie Sawyer and Carmel Hopkins for their guidance.

Acknowledgments

Photography provided by Tony Scodwell, Industrial Photographic, Tom Donoghue and Pablo Mason.

Synopsis and biography written by Carmel Hopkins.

TABLE CONTENTS

FOREWORD

(Editor's Note: Freelance writer Mike Henle underwent brain surgery to stop a seizure disorder at Scripps Green Hospital Dec. 6, 1994 in La Jolla, California. His book details a thirty-year illness, which was corrected by a surgical procedure at Scripps Green Hospital.)

For many years, I have been encouraged to write my own book. However, it wasn't until I had brain surgery, December 6, 1994, at Scripps Green Hospital in La Jolla, California, that my life changed enough to concentrate on such an awesome task.

There are countless people I'd like to thank for helping me create this book and the many thoughts that go with it. Needless to say, fighting chronic illness—caused by a mysterious disorder and compounded by heavy prescription drugs—is no easy task. I am here only because of the Good Lord, my family, my good friends and the people of Scripps Green Hospital.

True, I'm a fighter, and have been since the time that mosquito bit me when I was nine months old, infecting me with encephalitis. The sickness burned the right side of my brain, leaving me with a hounding seizure disorder. There have been a lot of troublesome times, but the unwillingness to give up was well worth it.

I finally found a doctor who would listen, Dr. Maung "Andy" Aung, a neurologist of Scripps Clinic. Together with neurosurgeon Dr. Thomas Waltz, Aung created an award-winning team, which literally changed my life.

You get so tired of being sick and especially having doctors refuse to listen to you. Dr. Aung listened when I told him I found my problem in a book in the library at the University of San Diego. He refused to give up, and with the help of Dr. Waltz and the staff of

Scripps Green Hospital, a huge war was won.

For thirty-seven years I was sick. I cannot state the number of times I felt like crawling in a hole because I was embarrassed by my medical problems. Nobody knew what was wrong, and quite honestly, there were times when I just didn't want to live anymore. It took that long to finally find someone who would not only listen, but also rewire a brain that had been badly hurt by seizures.

Finally, I'm free of prescription drugs and the side effects they leave. Yes, the whole battle was tough, but I'm here to tell you not to give up. The shackles have been taken off, and I'm on a roll now.

This is written for all of you who have had seizure disorders. Don't give up, because I'm living proof that you must be aggressive in your battle. Don't ever turn your back on your health problems, and most of all, find people like the ones who helped me get on my feet.

Take it from me when I tell you to get a second opinion. Question why you are taking a particular drug, and know the side effects. Get after it. Read books. Talk to friends and find someone who really cares.

It's so nice now to walk through a park without worrying about falling on my face. And it's wonderful to drive through the country, enjoying the beauty of the scenery.

My world has been opened up, and I can now reach my true potential because I'm free of a serious health problem. There was an answer out there, and I knew I had to find it. Like so many others, I had been told over the years that I could have other problems (like multiple sclerosis), but there was never an answer.

I can't tell you how many times I simply left the doctor, paid at the counter and headed for the pharmacy to load up on more prescription drugs. Getting off the drugs (such as phenobarbital) was perhaps one of the greatest fights of my life, and the freedom I now have is absolutely unbelievable.

Surgery was tough, but the addiction with the drugs was nearly unbearable. Once I finished the surgery, I had another battle in front of me in a struggle to wean myself from the drugs, which owned my life.

The most important fact is that I'm seizure free. Not one has occurred since the day before the surgery. Ten years later, I'm still amazed every time I think about the entire ordeal.

It is my understanding that seizures return in many cases. I feared that might happen for quite some time after the surgery, but never had to come to grips with such an ordeal, thank God.

This was more than life changing. It was a lifesaver. The seizure disorder probably would have taken me from this earth before my time. Worse yet, it could have resulted in someone else being hurt. No longer do my friends and family have to anguish at the sight of their loved one struggling to survive.

My life was a disaster, and I didn't even know it. I had learned to accept my seizure-ridden lifestyle, which would turn into chaos with every seizure. I didn't give much thought to a "normal" life until I actually was blessed with one.

If you're healthy, never take your good health for granted. And if you're sick, do something about it.

Take control of your life, as much as you can. I got my chance, and so can you.

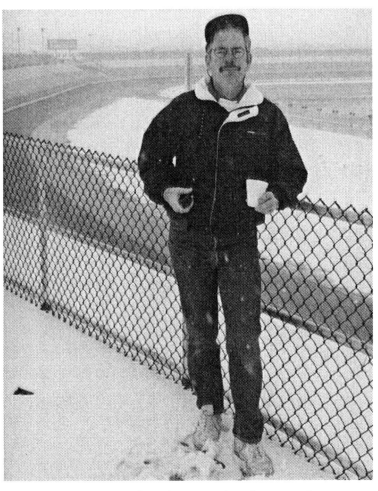

Here I am experiencing a pair of unusual moments in December of 1999 five years after the surgery: a day minus the threat of seizures and a snow storm at Las Vegas Motor Speedway.

CHAPTER 1

THE FIRST OF MANY SEIZURES

For some reason, that weekday afternoon in 1958 stands out in my mind as though it was yesterday. Even though it was almost forty years ago, I can still remember vividly what happened.

At the age seven, I was sitting home watching the *Art Linkletter Show* one afternoon while living in Carmel, California. I had just completed another day of school, and as usual, spent my time by myself at home after the bell had rung.

I always watched Linkletter when I was a young kid. There wasn't much to do in the afternoons other than play with my dog or watch television. The woods of Carmel didn't have many kids, and the schoolyard was usually empty. With that in mind, I just headed home with my dog, plopped myself down on the couch and watched television.

Linkletter was interviewing youngsters with that touch only he had. The room started going around in circles while I was lying on the couch. I suddenly experienced this rush of fear.

Now, almost four decades later, I'm starting to realize that first "spell" was the beginning of hundreds—and maybe even thousands—which I'd have. It caught me off-guard.

Quite frankly, I remember this rush of fear I experienced as the sensation raced through my head. I was sitting on the couch, and just sat there in an effort to regain my senses. Not sure what was taking place, I attempted to shake off what would eventually be diagnosed as a seizure.

I believe I eventually informed my parents of what had happened, and it wasn't long after that I was taken to Stanford Medical Center for tests. The tests were inconclusive, and the "funny feelings" which began on that weekday afternoon would eventually become more frequent.

As an adult, I think I know firsthand what little kids feel like when they're sick only to be told nothing is wrong. Quite honestly, I just learned to live with my disorder. In the long run, maybe it made me a better person, since I didn't complain about every ache and pain.

I didn't know how to explain what was happening. My dad looked at this sort of thing as "growing pains," something his own mother used to say about him when he was a little fella.

When petit mal or complex partial seizures hit, there was usually a strange aura that warned me something was wrong. While it's hard to explain, a sudden sensation came over me gaining intensity as the seconds went on. Sometimes the sensation would seem to end before the seizure gained strength. As I got older, I noticed the aura became stronger. There was generally no turning back once the aura started.

There is no explanation for why your face has gone blank and your speech is slurred. And in my particular case, that "funny feeling" I used to tell my mother about was something that I just learned to live with.

There was no telling when the room would start going around in circles again. But as time went on, I just continued to think everything was actually normal. Other people surely experienced such feelings, didn't they? I was just a little guy, not really sure what was going on and certain all this would end someday.

As we would later discover, the seizures were the result of encephalitis, which I had contacted when I was nine months old. I had apparently been bitten by a mosquito, which had transmitted the illness from a horse. I went into a coma for a week, and there was damage to the brain, the result of a high fever.

Little did we know that the illness several years prior would begin driving me into a real tailspin.

Chapter 2

That Horrible Needle

As a little guy, the seizures continued. But there never was an answer, just theories.

All I knew was that they were getting worse. They would strike at any time, whether I was in a deep sleep or standing in the outfield of a baseball game.

No one ever recognized the problem, primarily because I shrugged off what was happening on the outside. Inside, I was a nervous wreck once the aura started hoping to sidestep this strange sensation, but I knew the "spells" were getting worse.

I particularly remember one time when at the age of fourteen, I was playing baseball in Yuba City, California. The seizure hit and all I could do was hope no one would hit the ball to me. Standing there by myself in center field, I recall vividly trying to shake the feeling before I had to react to a fly ball or a ground ball.

It was 1965 and little did I know that it would take thirty more years of confusion to figure this out. I just kept fighting, giving the problem little thought. I continued to function, but it would take until I was in my mid-forties before I actually realized how difficult life had been at the time.

As a teenager, I didn't hit the ground, but my world was certainly going around in circles. For several minutes, I would feel disoriented and frightened. I'd dodge one bullet and get ready for another. The ice was getting thinner and the rope was beginning to tighten around my throat, although I really was unaware of the severity of the problem at the time.

And on a day in November 1966, the "funny feelings" came to a

17

head on the basketball court at Rancho High School in North Las Vegas. I was only fifteen at the time, and the problem wasn't going away.

I then began to experience double vision. I kept shaking my head, thinking the sensation would go away.

Then, someone passed me the ball. Before I knew it, the ball seemed to split in two and hit me. For several days, I continued to shake the double vision. But the problem was getting worse.

Because there were no noticeable effects from the spells, it was tough for my family to really react. In a matter of a minute or two, I was fine and we probably all looked at the episodes as my own version of "spacing out."

Unlike a bruise or a cut, there simply was no wound to treat. The entire experience was baffling to all of us because we couldn't pinpoint a particular area of concern.

When a car malfunctions, you replace the worn parts and keep going. And when the gas tank is low, you fill up and get on down the road. But what in the hell do you do after a person simply fades away? If I were fortunate enough to hide the spell, I'd simply go on with it. And if someone happened to notice, I struggled to explain what had taken place.

But in all honesty, none of us knew what to do. There weren't any broken parts to fix that we could determine. In looking back, it was almost like the computer system was going haywire and we hadn't yet entered the computer era.

Finally, I had had enough. My folks sent me to Dr. James Murphy at North Las Vegas Clinic. This old-time doctor with that cigarette hanging out of his mouth was the first man to finally get some sort of feel for this.

Murphy sat back in his chair, reading a book. After several minutes of intense reading, he determined that I had petit-mal epilepsy. He prescribed Dilantin, an anti-convulsant, and I began taking the drug three times a day. While the Dilantin came in capsules, the absolute worst taste came when one of the capsules opened in the mouth. The powder had a horribly bitter taste.

The Dilantin would eventually attack my liver more than twenty years later. Doctors would say that it was nerves, but medical tests would show the Dilantin was actually was attacking my liver. With my hectic schedule, I failed to have my blood level checked. The end result could have been deadly.

The problem didn't seem to get any better, though. And when we took the situation a step farther, I ran headlong into one of the most horrible medical procedures on earth.

In the 1960s before MRIs were first used, pneumoencephalograms were used to check for brain tumors. And while the MRI is a painless procedure where the patient is rolled into a long tube for x-rays, the pneumoenchephlogram proved to be nothing less than brutal.

It was explained to me that the pneumoencephalogram helped chart a possible tumor by first x-raying the brain. Then, doctors explained, it was necessary to dry up the brain cavities through something that would have to be considered about as terrifying as shock treatment.

Simply put, the procedure was a spinal tap. That in itself was bad enough.

Sitting on the edge of the table, I was told to put my head in a vice. The doctors said to move my head from side to side, because they were concerned that my spine would collapse during the procedure.

"Doc, I'm scared," I said, looking at a needle, which appeared to be twelve inches long.

"Good," the doctor said. "That means you're normal."

The physician deadened the area around the spine, and inserted the needle. That didn't hurt, but what would follow is something I'll never forget.

It was at that point that the brain cavity was filled with air. Up the spine went the air. And when it hit the brain, it was as though a balloon was about to pop. When the skull had received its air, I was rolled over to one side. More x-rays were taken and compared to the x-rays taken before the procedure. If the x-rays showed an abnormality in the brain, it was generally believed the patient had a tumor. No answers, but plenty of pain physically and emotionally. I had no tumor, but one helluva headache. And it would remain locked up in my head for at least two weeks.

One helluva lot of pain and the same "I dunno" look of the doctors. My God, there had to be some sort of answer to this mystery.

Chapter 3
They're Ruining My Career...

By the mid-1980s, I was in the middle of a sparkling career as a sportswriter with the *Las Vegas Review-Journal*, covering auto racing, University of Nevada, Las Vegas basketball and high school athletics.

My professional life was good, but my health was not good. I retained the belief that my illness would correct itself. Las Vegas had been good to a kid from Northern California, but the medical problems persisted. I had moved south, found a career in journalism and was happy with the changes in my life.

I missed the greenery of Northern California, but loved being a sportswriter. By the time I was fifteen, I was covering professional boxing, high school athletics, and anything else that came along. I wasn't afraid of deadlines, thrived on covering sports, and hit the ground running in Las Vegas on a cold November day.

When I entered Rancho High School in 1966, I needed one class. Journalism 101 was there, I took the bait and off I went. I couldn't imagine getting paid for doing something that I loved. I spent so much time at the *Las Vegas Sun* doing research on high school basketball that I was asked to cover high school basketball games for $1.25 an hour.

I was in high gear, never missing a shift. I covered the Strip Fight of the Week at the old Silver Slipper in a smoke-filled room that was formerly a bingo hall and moved to the *Las Vegas Review-Journal* as a senior in high school covering high school athletics.

I only looked at the clock to make sure I was going to meet deadline. I wasn't a big fan of the desert, but was so busy that I never paid too much attention to the scenery. Things were going well, and when I wasn't covering sports, I was busing dishes at the Mint Hotel.

However, it was in 1978 that I had been introduced to the Big Daddy of all scares – a grand-mal seizure. The activity in the brain was obviously getting worse. As I was told, a scar on the side of the brain—the result of a high fever when I was an infant—was growing. Thus, so was the target. For some reason, I kept waking up in the middle of the night with horrible headaches. I literally felt as though someone had taken a sledgehammer to the top of my head. No aspirin could provide relief when the top of my skull literally felt as though it was going to explode.

I kept wondering if the pneumoencephalogram had left serious damage. The headaches were just like the ones I had when they sent that rush of air up my spine and into my skull.

While I noticed that the frequency was continuing, I also realized that my sleep habits were changing. You see, you don't sleep well when it feels like a stick of TNT has gone off between your ears.

Anywhere. Anytime.

But surely, these things would go away, I kept telling myself. Little did I know this was only getting worse, and while doctors kept prescribing drugs, matters continued to worsen.

I could deal with the petit-mal seizures, and was confident that my life would hold up okay.

Then, in the middle of the night in 1978, all hell broke loose. I suddenly awoke to this horrible headache, which sent me spinning around the room. My wife of six years, Carmen, was pregnant with our second child at the time, when she heard me gnashing my teeth. She frantically tried to hold me in bed, as my body stiffened. Without a doubt, in the nearly ten years since our first date, Carmen had seen the situation getting worse as the blank stares suddenly gravitated to full-blown grand-mal seizures.

I remember nothing other than awakening to the horrible headache. The next thing I knew, there were people standing over me, and Carmen was crying hard.

"You've had a seizure," she cried. "We need to get you to the hospital now."

I was scared because of the unknown. I had no idea what was wrong or what had happened. My family was scared because of what they had seen. It wasn't pretty, and everyone was confused and frightened.

A trip to the hospital, and I was shot up with medication and sent home. There were no solutions, no answers. Surely this was only a bad day. Little did I know that I had many more bad days in front of me.

Chapter 4
The Fast Lane With Plenty of Yellow Flags

Las Vegas, which gives many people a lease on life, was giving me my continued chance in the 1980s. While my health was still on a roller coaster ride, Las Vegas began to focus its attention on big-time motor sports, something I had always dreamed of covering.

Caesars Palace, a plush resort which seemed to lead the world in blockbuster events, announced it was going to present a Formula One Grand Prix on the grounds of its parking lot. I was about to cover a massive event in a city that never sleeps.

I couldn't have been more at home. I had so much going for me in journalism that I really didn't have time to worry about my health. I was still convinced that the mysterious problem would magically clear itself up.

The petit-mal seizures continued, but I hid most of them. My family and good friends would notice that blank look on my face, and know I was having another, but most people never gave them a second thought. I kept hiding from my problems, but another setback was just around the corner.

While the seizures continued, I tried hard to keep taking my medicine. However, nothing seemed to work. I was confused, scared, and feeling as though my life was a big time bomb.

There was also a hidden concern on my part that I did not share with anyone. While I was expected to take prescription drugs, I had seen the abuse of prescription drugs when I was a kid. My mother had been addicted to various prescription drugs and the thought that the same could happen to me was a huge worry. I kept taking the Dilantin, but not without reservations. I had witnessed some very difficult times when I was a kid and the thought of having to count on drugs to survive was a burden I did not want to shoulder for the rest of my life. I was to take the medicine three times a day. I had always been active and remembering to stop and take medicine was a hassle. However, I tried hard to follow the schedule.

But nothing was working. We added more drugs, this time phenobarbital, tiny pills that were to help stop the seizures. No matter what I took, the seizures continued. I wasn't big on alcohol and lived a clean life.

Worse yet, every drug had a side effect. Dilantin made the gums swell and as I would later discover, it can attack the liver. Phenobarbital leaves a person feeling sluggish, and that was tough for a peppy person like myself. When a seizure would hit, my loved ones would remind me that I needed to take my medication. I attempted to take the pills with me so as not to forget them. I'd always nodded and agreed to take the medicine, but most people probably knew of my concerns. I just wanted to live life without medicine or seizures.

My stomach had begun to hurt for some reason, but I tried not to pay any attention to the pain. My weight was dwindling and everyone was concerned. I maintained an attitude that things would change for the better.

Little did I know that things were only getting worse. I kept my drag race pace and was enjoying my career. My career as a sportswriter kept my mind off my own health problems.

I was hiding the problem, as best as I could. When the seizures would hit, I'd struggle to keep my head up and sometimes begin limping on my left leg. I'd take a deep breath and keep going. If I were by myself, I'd cease what I was doing for a minute and catch my breath.

As bad as things were, I kept making the best of things. Covering high school athletics and auto racing was very enjoyable, but those close to me knew that things weren't going well.

I kept searching for help groups that concentrated on the health problems I was going through. However, there was no help in Las Vegas and doctors seemed to shrug their shoulders when I walked through the door.

It was a massive guessing game, but I had never been one to give up hope. I kept thinking another seizure was my last. "I'm just having a bad day," I'd say to myself. "Things are certain to get better and we'll get this thing figured out."

CHAPTER 5
THEY'RE GETTING WORSE

It's funny when you're sick all of the time you really don't know there is such a thing as a good day. While all of your days are generally bad ones, there is no reason to feel that you're anything other than normal. So, as time went on, I just kept thinking my "normal" life was something that I had to deal with. But as time went on, my head began to hurt more often. I had no answers, just more theories. And every time I got my hopes up, my world came crashing down on me again. As I continued to fumble around, I discovered that the activity in the brain was getting worse, apparently because the scar on the right side of the brain was growing.

This was the ideal example of learning by the seat of your pants, I guessed, but I just continued to figure things out a little more every day.

I kept waking up in the middle of the night with horrible headaches. The drugs kept coming and the illness kept getting worse. It was a race between the drugs and the seizures as to which would do me in first. My wife and our children all saw things getting worse. *My God*, I thought. I wasn't drowning myself in alcohol or illegal drugs. I didn't want anything to do with this damned disorder, which was slowly but surely killing me. The drugs seemed to be eating away at my liver and kidneys and hurting every part of my body.

Working in the newspaper business, I arose early every morning to arrive at work at six. I loved the business, and was eager to get to work every morning. Frankly, I was always thankful for the opportunity to work at the *Las Vegas Review-Journal*, because it afforded me the chance to follow a career that I absolutely loved.

Work was fine, but my health was going downhill fast. Carmen

27

began to notice that I was gnashing my teeth more often in my sleep, a sure sign that something was definitely wrong. I would later discover that the brain's ability to function—and most importantly to remember things—was being hampered by the scar above the right ear.

I'd wake up in the middle of the night, with my head going in circles. It seemed as though the attacks took place while I was in a very deep sleep.

We had continued to fight the confusing health problem, and I dug deeper and deeper for answers. Unfortunately, it just didn't seem as though everyone else was digging as hard as I was.

Once our second child was born, we decided to head for Dairy Queen for a celebration. With a three-year-old in the car and a brand new baby next to him as they sat in the truck, I ordered what I thought was our big celebration.

While standing in line, the room began to go around in circles. I again thought this would straighten itself out. A short time later, I was on the floor in the middle of a grand-mal seizure.

The paramedics were called and my frantic family watched, as I worked through the seizure. A man grabbed a brush, placed it in my mouth and tried to make sure I didn't swallow my tongue. One of my teeth was chipped, and I felt horrible. Nauseated, I struggled to tell everyone that I was fine. Just give me a little more time to be by myself.

The paramedics decided it was better to get me to the hospital, so they rushed my family into the ambulance. Confused and scared, I struggled to figure out why this was happening.

It may have been that trip to the hospital that really encouraged me to get a handle on this. Again, more drugs and little answers, but this time it was even worse.

The doctor informed my wife and mother-in-law that I was simply stressed out. No big deal, just take me home and let me relax.

Shoot him up and get him out of here.

Take a number, please.

Next.

Chapter 6
The Downfall in Long Beach

The petit-mal seizures continued to come in clusters for quite some period of time. I felt I could handle them fine. It was just the big ones that really worried me.

I was thriving in my career as a sports writer, having the time of my life. I had been assigned to cover the Long Beach Grand Prix in 1982, when another chapter in my life was written.

I had taken my wife with me because her uncle lived in Long Beach. We had figured that the trip would be fun, since we could combine pleasure with business.

I eagerly headed for the pressroom of the Long Beach Grand Prix. The setting was awesome, considering the backdrop of the city. The noise of the cars completed the atmosphere and I was in hog heaven.

Auto racing and journalism were the ideal package for me. I was getting to travel, and was readying myself for the Caesars Palace Grand Prix, which had been planned for an area off the Las Vegas Strip.

As I walked to the pressroom, I noticed the feeling of a seizure. It was warm outside, and these kinds of things happened when there was significant heat. But while the dizziness started, I assured myself that I would just shake this one off. It wasn't to be that easy, however.

As my head continued to swirl, I noticed that this one was not going away. All of a sudden, I heard a woman ask me if I was okay. And that was it. Down I went in full view of hundreds of people. I blacked out cold, only to awaken in the emergency room of a Long Beach hospital. Before I knew it, Carmen was running into the room crying.

I had written her uncle's phone number down on a notepad. In the eyes of the paramedics, I was simply a John Doe in deep trouble. However, when the phone number rang at my wife's uncle's home, she knew immediately what was wrong. Call it a sixth sense. There had been trouble at the Long Beach Grand Prix, and it wasn't because Mario Andretti had crashed.

I had crashed badly. And again, there was no answer. I went back and lay down, only to arise a short time later. A call to the *Las Vegas Review-Journal* news desk let my employer know that I had just collapsed.

Nobody knew why. But surely, this had to be the last of the big-time seizures I thought. For some reason, I always thought this one seizure was to be my last. As was the case with every other seizure, the doctors in Long Beach had no answers.

I slept for a few hours at my wife's uncle's house, washed my face, and got back after it. I was groggy, but that was to be expected, we were told.

The petit-mal seizures were mild enough to live with, but the grand mals sent a startling reminder that this was no game. They hit hard, and left me feeling punch drunk and embarrassed, wondering what had happened.

CHAPTER 7
THAT DAMNED LITTLE
MOSQUITO

While I was trying to live by the belief that you outgrew epilepsy, I was only dreaming. It seemed that the older I got, the worse the seizures became. Once it was determined that an illness I had when I was an infant was the root of the problem, we began to understand why the seizures continued.

When I was nine months old, my mother and father had been playing cards with friends when I apparently went into a convulsion. A mosquito that carried the encephalitis virus had apparently bitten me. I went into a coma for a week, but everyone back then apparently believed time would pass and so would the illness.

Little did we all know that the infection had burned the right side of the brain. As we would discover in my thirties, the disease hadn't disappeared at all. It was just getting stronger. Even with careful diets suggested by some doctors, we had all discovered that the disorder owned me. The little, tiny scar on the right side of the brain was simply getting bigger as the brain continued to grow. According to what I was told, the brain reaches its full size at the age of thirty.

So the little tiny scar left by the encephalitis had grown with the size of the brain. To make a long story short, the bigger the scar the bigger the chance of seizures.

One more theory, but at least I began to understand this disorder. I knew it wasn't my imagination, as I would discover in my readings. It was epilepsy that was playing havoc with my life, although one Las Vegas neurologist theorized that I was in the beginning stages of multiple sclerosis.

I walked out of the doctor's office, and kept searching. He was wrong, as we would later discover and I was happy that I had trusted my own gut feeling.

The seizures were not going away, and the kids began to notice dear old Dad in his failings. As soon as a seizure would begin, they'd notice. I couldn't hide them any longer and it just baffled me that everyone noticed so quickly.

If I were in the middle of a conversation with someone, I'd simply walk away. People shook their heads, wondering if they had said something wrong. It was embarrassing to say the least, but I just learned to live with the hassles of the disease.

Once everyone understood what was taking place, they'd try to help. However, I kept wondering if I wasn't the only person on earth with this baffling disorder. As I would later discover, many people suffered from the disorder and like me, most didn't know where to turn.

We had begun experimenting with more prescription drugs. Nothing worked, though. Mysoline made me violently ill and Dilantin had attacked the liver. Tegretol leaves you nervous and with dry mouth. I continued taking phenobarbital, which I would later discover was horribly addictive.

When the Dilantin attacked the liver, I was immediately ordered to get off it. The lump under my rib cage was the result of the Dilantin, which had begun to poison the organ. A lethal level of the drug had sent warning signals, which were discovered after blood work was ordered.

We continued to try finding something that would work. Nothing was effective, and everything had a side affect. Once the side effect would start, I was told just to be patient. But I absolutely hated the drugs and the problems they brought with them.

CHAPTER 8
WORD HAS SPREAD

By the mid-1980s, word had spread about the problems I was having with the seizure disorder. On one hand, I didn't want anyone knowing about my woes. But on the other hand, I'm glad now that someone spread the word. You see, it was back during this period of time that a Las Vegas insurance salesman named John Marxen called me one day at the *Las Vegas Review-Journal.*

Marxen didn't call much, but we had mutual friends in John and Mary Keiser of Las Vegas. The Keisers had apparently said something to Marxen about my problem and I will thank them until the day I die for that blessing.

I had met Marxen through the Keisers, and had done a story on his youthful son, who was quite a soccer player. I made a star out of Marxen's son in the story I wrote, and we became friends.

"Herkie" Marxen would go on to become a star kicker, both in soccer and football. His dad would ultimately lead me to a new life, one where I was free of a dreaded illness that owned every move I made.

"Henle, I understand you're having Marxen problems," was the greeting from John Marxen.

I really didn't quite know what to make of the statement. But the truth of the matter was that Marxen was about to point the way to a man who would literally turn my life around nearly a decade later.

Enter a little guy from Burma named Dr. M. H. Aung.

"Henle, I'm telling you," Marxen said. "You've got to go see Dr. Aung. This man is the greatest. I've had the same problems as you, and he literally turned me around."

Dr. Aung was not present when I finally visited Scripps in the late

1980s. He was out of town and the people of Scripps forwarded me to a neurologist named Dr. Jack Sipe.

Dr. Sipe agreed that there was a problem, but determined that I should start taking a drug called Tegretol. *Here we go again*, I thought. *Pour more poison down my throat and we'll see what happens.*

I pleaded with Dr. Sipe to find an answer and asked if there was a chance that surgery would end my problems. He said he feared surgery, since it was so close to the optic nerve. Surgery, he said, was way too dangerous. I was not convinced that he was right, but headed back to Las Vegas to resume my life.

Even though Sipe was against surgery, I had reached a point in my life where taking a chance wasn't something that I was afraid of anymore. What the hell, every day was a chance at this rate.

I took Sipe's advice and began taking the Tegretol. However, two days later, I knew there was another problem. After determining that dry mouth was a serious consequence of taking the drug, I was removed from it.

My stomach had really begun to hurt from all the medication and the turmoil. So, while I was fighting epilepsy with the drugs, I was fighting the drugs with stomach medicine. It had become a vicious circle, chasing one woe with another.

I was so tired of people telling me that I looked awful. But the truth of the matter was that I was looking bad. Some voiced concern that I had cancer, while others figured I was just out of gas.

One doctor in particular advised me, "You're going to have to give up the job or learn to deal with the stress."

Figuring stress was the problem, I finally announced in November of 1989 that I was leaving my position as real estate editor of the *Las Vegas Review-Journal*. It was a very difficult decision, but I felt that due to my health's steady decline, I would try anything to get well.

So in December, about three hundred of us gathered in the dance hall of the Gold Coast Hotel and Casino and I moved on with my life. The Randy Anderson Band, an entertaining country western band, played the music and I danced away twenty-one years of memories from the *Las Vegas Review-Journal*. I agonized over the idea of leaving a writing career, but was literally at my wit's end. I didn't know what it would be like to start another business, but dove into it headfirst.

Marxen and I stayed in touch periodically, and always talked about my health. We never saw one another without Marxen asking me if I had gone to meet with Dr. Aung yet. Tenacious, Marxen would not back down, and he continually swore to me that Andy Aung was the best in the business for seizure disorders.

But through it all, the call from John Marxen proved to be a very important twist in my desire to get well. It had actually spelled a turn in my life. There wasn't to be a quick turnaround, but a path had been bladed.

I didn't get to Dr. Aung the first time, but on the plane home I knew I was going back. While it took awhile to understand that, I had actually started to get a handle on the seizure disorder. Besides, Scripps Hospital, situated just north of San Diego, was near the ocean. I loved the environment. In my opinion, if I had to be sick, there could be no better place to recover than near the ocean. And while there wasn't an answer yet, I felt that I had started the journey to recovery.

While I had left Scripps the first time somewhat discouraged, I knew that I would return. The scenery was beautiful, the people of the hospital seemed to care, and I wasn't giving up.

CHAPTER 9

MY CAREER AND HEALTH ARE GOING IN OPPOSITE DIRECTIONS

My life as a freelance writer had actually started to prosper in 1990 as I picked up various accounts. I purchased a lap top computer, hit the streets running, and attempted to put my health problems behind me. I could run, but I couldn't hide. No broken-field runner can escape the threat of seizures, and I was discovering that quickly.

In addition to writing public relations releases for several clients, I was also working at a racetrack. With the track and real estate-oriented clients, I stayed extremely busy in my first year of serving as an independent businessman.

I had never handled my own books before, and had never invoiced anyone before. I came up with the name "The Idea Co." and churned out press releases with a spirited dedication. Things were actually going well and I was adjusting to the rigors of running my own business. I had always wondered what it would be like to be my own man in charge of my own destiny, and I was quickly learning the ropes.

There were taxes to pay and there were invoices to send. While I was scared, I seemed to thrive on the activity. But while I was running Mach 1 in business, I was also unable to rid myself of the health problems.

Just when I hit high gear, the seizure disorder would raise its head again. While the tonicoclonic seizures seemed to have subsided, the petit mals were getting stronger. That blank stare associated with the seizure was becoming more prevalent.

Additionally, each time a seizure would hit, my left side would begin to go limp. If I was walking, I would droop to the left side issuing a signal to everyone around me that something was suddenly wrong.

I kept thinking constantly about what Jack Sipe had said about the surgery. The optic nerve may have been too close, but the seizures were taking more and more control of my life.

There were many longs hours affiliated with everything I had going on in business. The seizures were hitting all times of the day and night. When I became fatigued, they'd hit with more strength.

And when seizures hit, they came in droves. It was like being attacked by an army of demons. One would hit and a few hours later, another would take its toll.

Seizures in the middle of the night seemed to be more common than ever before. I'd wake up feeling as though a stick of dynamite had gone off in my head, leaving me confused and worried.

I could go weeks without a seizure. If one hit, I knew I was in for a few days of unsettled times, since the attacks came in droves. Just when I'd begin to relax, I'd get hit again. Most times I was able to hide the immediate problem. But the long-range woes were tearing my stomach up and wearing me very thin.

I was determined to get back to Scripps. If that didn't work, I had read that the University of Minnesota Medical Department specialized in the treatment of seizures. And if that didn't work, Germany's medical technology was highly regarded. There was no limit to what could be done, as far as I was concerned.

I wasn't taking "I dunno" for an answer anymore. Getting well had become my passion.

The years 1990-94 were a blur, as I continued to run my business. I had discovered the money affiliated with advertising; and marveled at the radio and television businesses.

Epilepsy support groups were virtually nonexistent, but I did begin hearing more about others with the problem. In particular, a television report told of a young woman who had gone to UCLA for a surgical procedure to eliminate a seizure disorder. Sue Mortal, who

I would later meet, beat epilepsy with the surgery and I was certain that I, too, could get hold of this. Ironically, Sue's best friend was the mother of our son's best buddy.

The skies began to open up. I received more reason to have hope, since others were finding the reason. Scripps and UCLA were both within three hundred miles and Germany wasn't out of the question either.

The business was continuing to grow, but so was the health problem. I refused to give up on both of them and stayed busy reading books and talking to people.

Sue Mortal's story absolutely fascinated me. And the fact that we actually had a mutual friend was incredible. Sue turned her life around and I could do the same I insisted. A report on NBC illustrated a marvelous story about a young woman who had finally gotten her life together thanks to the surgery.

In the meantime, I kept taking the phenobarbital and whatever else was expected to end my seizure disorder. But the drugs weren't working and we all knew it.

CHAPTER 10

CALLING TO THE HEAVENS FOR HELP

In the fall of 1994, our family had experienced a tough year. It was in 1993 that we had purchased a lot to build our own home. At the same time, my mother-in-law had been diagnosed with pancreatic cancer. We plunged headlong into the development of our home and broke ground a short time before Arline Rivero died in April of that year.

We really bit off more than we could chew. But thinking that the construction of the home would soothe our sorrow, we kicked our lives into full gear. And it was about that time that we were about to get hammered again. The seizures began taking their toll once again, just as we began construction on our home. When the heat hit during the middle of the summer, all hell broke loose in more ways than one.

While working to clean up the backyard, I suddenly felt myself going down. Our middle son, Joe, came to my rescue. He led me to cooler temperatures and assured me that I'd be okay.

The intensity of the seizures was beginning to become worse than they had been before. I just kept my head up as much as possible.

Then, on one hot afternoon, the roof began to cave in. My neighbor, UNLV baseball coach Rod Soesbe, saw me going down and called for my wife. I could hear Rod calling to me and I could hear him calling for Carmen. But the funny thing about it was that I could not respond. I felt helpless, almost paralyzed. Soesbe would later tell my father-in-law that it appeared that I was looking up to the heavens for help. Little did he know that he was probably right. Call it a move of desperation or a simple call for help. It's funny how things work out sometimes, but this honestly felt as though I was looking for an extra bit of help. In my shoes, I needed everything I could get my hands on.

The seizures had become like lightning rods running through my head every time they went off. My left side was starting to give way, and those around me could see that I was limping more following a seizure. I told my wife that the seizures actually felt like strokes. I told her I was heading for Scripps and this time I was going to get hold of Dr. Aung.

I've never really given much thought to my tenacity, but my dad once said I was like a bulldog. Once I got my teeth into something, I wouldn't give up. Perhaps the name "Mad Dog," given to me at the *Review-Journal*, was fitting.

So when Rod Soesbe had to pick me up in the backyard in 1994, I had finally had enough. I was determined that I had been beaten up enough. Like a badly beaten prizefighter, sick and tired of being humiliated in front of people, I climbed from the earth, looked to the heavens, and said I wasn't taking any more of this. Whatever devil was beating me up, I had taken his last punch. This wasn't going away, and taking prescription medication certainly wasn't helping things either.

I called Scripps Hospital again, and this time I wanted to see Dr. Aung. I don't know why I was so sure that he could fix the problem, but I wasn't going to see anyone else. There had been too many dead-end roads, too many people shrugging their shoulders. I wasn't taking it anymore.

I called Scripps and made the appointment to see Dr. Aung. I then followed with another call to make my room reservations at the Torrey Pines Inn next to the hospital.

CHAPTER 11

LIVING WITH THAT CONSTANT FEAR

I often wondered if building our dream home wasn't a huge mistake. Our family had experienced such tough times when my mother-in-law was diagnosed with cancer in early 1994. But, we always knew that Arline Rivero wanted us to have the best. She loaned us the money to purchase our first house in 1972, when we purchased a tiny, but warm twelve hundred square-foot three-bedroom home in an older neighborhood called Twin Lakes in Las Vegas.

So, when it was determined that Arline wasn't doing well at all, we pressed on. We had to be persistent and live our dream. "Follow your heart" had become one of my favorite phrases, so when questioning a decision, I leaned on the line.

I will never forget the sight of Carmen sitting across from the table of the builder, pushing the plans toward him and giving him the go-ahead to begin construction of our home.

I looked back so many times and said that we took on way too much at the time. We broke ground on the home in April, as Arline sat in the car too sick to have a sip of champagne with us. She was able to see us launch our big home, only to pass away a short time later.

But while this was all completely too tough to understand at the time, building the home was good for us. And it was actually the turning point in my life, because it literally forced me to the ground for the last time.

To borrow a line from the song "The Weight" by The Band, I had pulled into town and felt about "half-past dead." I had carried this load way too long, and so had my family. Seizures were restricting me from doing what I loved most, because I never knew when they'd hit.

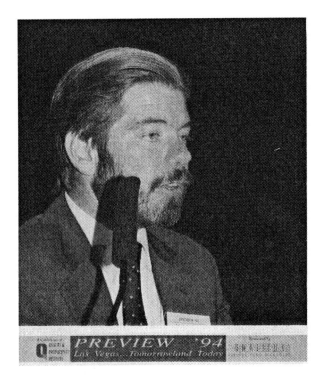

In December of 1993, I am shown speaking to a crowd of about 2,000 at Preview '94 at the Mirage Hotel. Little did anyone know that behind the microphone was a man who constantly worried about having a seizure. Thankfully, that part of my life is behind me now.

As a guest speaker at Preview '94 at the Mirage Hotel, I gave a speech to a group of more than one thousand people in December of 1993. The speech was about building our own home and the audience was impressed. Little did anyone know that I was terrified that I'd collapse in full view of everyone.

I had done a live television interview and given speeches and every time I was terrified. During one live television interview in an early-morning newscast, I felt myself slipping into a seizure. I attempted to hold my composure, knowing that a seizure on live television was unforgiving.

This wasn't an interview when someone could immediately yell to "cut." I regained my composure, thanked the heavens that I had been able to pull myself together, and realized that I had dodged another bullet. But I was getting so tired of the constant yellow flags of my life. I refused to give up living my life although I constantly felt as though I had a gun stuck to the side of my head.

After the television interview, I called home to ask my wife if she had noticed anything strange about my composure. Although she could usually catch the beginning of the seizure, she had missed this one. However, I didn't miss it. The close call left me weak and worried.

CHAPTER 12

THE CHAPTER OF MY RECOVERY

I checked into the Torrey Pines Inn near San Diego, and thought I'd head for the University of San Diego Medical Library across the street.

I had been searching books long and far for an answer to my problem for a long time, but this was one trip that I'll never forget for as long as I live.

I wandered over to the library, a beautiful facility with enough books to make you dizzy. As odd as it may sound, I was being attracted to this library. I had never been much of a spiritual person before, but this time there was a reason for me to be at this library at this time. I went to the computer to look up a book on stroke disorders. There must have been fifty books about strokes and I chose one.

I headed for the books, not really knowing how to look up the book I had found. But I kept searching until I found a book about strokes and the rest is history. Pulling the book off the shelf, I went to the back to see if there was anything on seizures. There was a listing about seizures and I kept looking. It was then that my heart jumped and I honestly felt as though I had been overcome. In the book I read that those who suffered from encephalitis as infants may later suffer from seizure disorders.

Call it "Divine Intervention," if you'd like. I was being affected spiritually. I suddenly had goose bumps on my arms. Standing in the library, I felt as though I had risen three feet. God was leading me down the right path, and I suddenly I was finding answers. I could not put the book down. Good Lord, there it was! Surely, this would lead me down the right path to recovery. I tried not to get too excited, but I couldn't help but have more hope. I went back to my room and went to bed, excited that I'd have an answer to this problem. Little did I know that what I had found in the book at the University of San Diego Medical Library was about to change my life. It hadn't taken another bottle of pills to solve my problem. It just took a good book and a little help from the Good Lord. I had the feeling and was sure some doctor was bound to have the cure. Little did I know how right I was.

Almost like a little kid who had found that great gift under a Christmas tree, I almost wanted to embrace this book. I put it back on the shelf, headed back for the Torrey Pines Inn and lay my head down on the pillow.

CHAPTER 13
THE LITTLE GUY WITH THE ANSWER

I'm usually early for my appointments, and I climbed out of bed to see Dr. Aung the next morning. I felt newly inspired. I checked into Scripps Hospital, asked for Dr. Aung's office and headed for my appointment.

Once inside my room, I began really wondering what Dr. Aung would look like. I suddenly had this freshly found hope. In walked a little man with a slight smile. It was Dr. Aung, and we began the usual exchange of question and answers. I explained that I was having trouble with seizures and they weren't getting any better. I hesitated to mention what I had found in the book the night before. Surely, I had no idea what I was talking about, I thought. *Just let him do his job and we'll go on with this.*

But something caused me say, "Dr. Aung, I know that I don't know anything about the medical profession, but I found something in a book last night that may help us figure out what is the matter."

Dr. Aung listened to me. I could tell that he was sincerely interested in what I was about to say. I had a sense that the man from Burma really cared and I hadn't even been in his office five minutes.

In nearly every hospital in the country, doctors are too busy. Without realizing it, they're running from one patient to another giving out prescriptions without even thinking. But Dr. Aung wasn't the traditional doctor of today's busy medical profession. He had a unique manner to him. I didn't feel as though I was wasting his time. After so many years of "I dunno" answers, he had a refreshing and professional manner. From that first appointment, I felt a sense of confidence. There was no rush-rush personality. He didn't move quickly and I could tell he wanted to hear my story.

"I found in a book last night that infants who have encephalitis can later suffer from seizure disorders," I said. "I'm sure no expert about this, but could this be the reason for my problem?"

Dr. Aung looked at me and said, "That may be. We're going to find out what is wrong."

Good Lord, I thought. *This man really cares about me. He's listening to what I have to say.*

"Okay, so now what's next?" I asked.

"We're going to put you through a series of tests," he responded. "We will find out what is wrong."

Dr. Aung explained that each test was a step to another. The first step was a MRI, of which I had many. I would be placed in a tube, and pictures of the brain would be taken. We would then follow with an EEG and finally a neuropsychological exam. The three procedures would take about three weeks to complete. I couldn't wait to get the reservations made this time.

Dr. Aung was so calm and so certain in his explanation. It took all of five minutes to figure out what we were going to do next.

CHAPTER 14

"THERE IT IS."

Both the EEG and the MRI are painless procedures. The only thing that bothered me about the many MRIs was the awful fear that I'd begin to choke in the middle of one of the procedures. I had begun noticing that seizures led to my choking. Lying on your back in this tunnel was no place to have a seizure, I had feared.

The MRI is conducted in a long tube-like mechanism. You are rolled into the tube, and state-of-the-art equipment takes pictures of your body to measure for problems. But that fear that I'd go into a seizure while in the middle of the tube was something that really frightened me. I kept telling myself that this would be a horrible way to die. It was easy to get claustrophobia while being stuck in that tube, and I continually concentrated to make sure I was swallowing properly.

A short time after the MRI, I headed for Dr. Aung's office.

"There it is," he said, pointing to one of several x-rays on the light bar. I immediately began to wonder if I had a brain tumor.

"What are you talking about?" I asked, since I knew absolutely nothing about what I was looking at.

"There is a scar on the right side of the brain," Dr. Aung said, pointing to a tiny dark mark on the x-ray. "It is the result of a high fever, and that may very well be what's causing your problems."

Remembering the phrase "persistence, persistence, persistence,"I immediately asked Dr. Aung if we could get this thing with surgery. However, I had doubts that he'd look at this possibility with a favorable outlook, considering that Jack Sipe had refused to take it to the next step.

"The damage has showed up on two tests," he explained. "There is a chance that we could do surgery, but you'll need one more test to see for sure."

Hey, just point the way. Where's my next stop?

Dr. Aung informed me that I still needed to have the neuropsychological exam. I had no clue what that entailed, but I did know that I wasn't giving up – and frankly, Dr. Aung wasn't about to back away either.

In auto racing terms, we were heading for the straightaway. The green flag was becoming more and more clear and we weren't about to pull our foot off of the accelerator yet.

CHAPTER 15
THE NEXT STEP

I had been sick for so many years that it really didn't make any difference to me what we needed to do. All I knew was that the book told us one thing, and Dr. Aung apparently found the evidence. With the surgery now becoming more of a possibility, I began to get my hopes up. I had begun to lose my will to live, and this couldn't go on any longer. Over and over again, I kept asking myself if living was worth it anymore.

Had it not been for my family, I would have given up long before. They were always there to pick me up from the canvas, and that is something I will remember until my dying day.

"There are three steps to determining whether or not you will be a candidate for surgery," Dr. Aung said. "Next week, we need you back for a neuropsychological exam, and that should tell us for sure."

By this time, I was nearly desperate to try anything. So, when I heard we were two-thirds of the way home, I wasn't about to back away.

The next week I arrived to meet with Dr. Jacobson, who would reveal some very fascinating problems about the brain through an intense three and a half hour question and answer session. A neuropsychological exam is a very friendly, but challenging ordeal. The psychologist told me stories, and showed me a set of blocks that I was asked to put together.

And it was then that I discovered why I had done so poorly when it came time to take exams. One year of college, and I was out on the streets trying to make a living, because I simply couldn't remember anything I had read in a book or heard in a classroom.

When the test was given, I generally finished low. Little did I know that the brain disorder was apparently causing me havoc through my entire life.

I couldn't repeat a story told me without missing one element or another. And I couldn't properly match figures after seeing them on previous pages.

Dr. Jacobson gave me a set of blocks, and I failed that portion of the exam so badly that he responded with, "I know what I'm going to give you for Christmas. You need practice."

Dr. Jacobson was a very unassuming individual. He made me feel comfortable from the time I sat down in his office. There was no problem feeling confident with him, and when he spoke, I was certain he knew what he was talking about. "Your results are revealing a problem on the right side of the brain," he explained. "The way you answer the questions are showing that."

Then, Dr. Jacobson really brought light to the problem. "It is a real tribute to you that you have been able to make a living as a journalist," he said. "There seems to be a big problem with your ability to remember."

For thirty years, I had simply thought I was not a very intelligent person. I accepted that philosophy and just worked harder.

"You know, now that you say that, I've always had to either use a tape recorder or take notes on the computer," I responded, almost in a sense of amazement.

"I can tell you this," Dr. Jacobson said. "You had better be thankful for the creation of the computer. I don't know what you would have done without it."

Now that I look back, there is a real sense of accomplishment in knowing that I had never made any crucial mistakes as a journalist. Among my writings have been four articles in the real estate section of the *New York Times*.

To be honest, I wanted to cry for a pair of reasons. First, I was proud of myself for refusing to give up. And finally, there again seemed to be light at the end of the tunnel. I was going to whip this thing, no matter what it took.

Little did I know that the biggest hurdle of all was yet to come.

Dr. Jacobson, by telling me that people had been cured of epilepsy through surgery, had created the final opinion. The information would be forwarded to Dr. Thomas Waltz, a neurosurgeon at Scripps Hospital.

CHAPTER 16
FOR THE FIRST TIME, FEAR SETS IN

I have always loved having my own office. The ability to get away from the hubbub has been good for me, and I love being able to turn on a radio and concentrate on something uninterrupted.

But never in my life have I ever seen an office like that of Dr. Thomas Waltz, a man who is on the board of directors of Scripps Hospital. When my wife and I were escorted into Dr. Waltz's office, I still had doubt in my mind. But once I looked out that big window in Dr. Waltz's office, there was that big, beautiful Pacific Ocean staring me in the face again.

The ocean is so soothing. I have always been able to relax by the sea and this was one time when I needed a deep level of relaxation. The sight had carried me through some very tough times, especially during the period of my life when I was searching for the answer to my health problem.

When I walked into Dr. Waltz's office, my arms softened. I just relaxed, even though I knew this wasn't going to be easy. And it seemed only fitting that the sight of the ocean should actually begin a meeting that would pave the way to my new life.

Dr. Waltz was gracious, and as usual, I wasn't scared. After all, I had been through these meetings so many times before, and I was sure I would simply be told there was nothing that could be done. But I was in for a powerful surprise. Dr. Waltz was a very calm man, someone who seemed to have a grasp on my predicament. For some reason, a doctor without an answer shows that in his face. But Dr.

Waltz had a look that carried promise.

"Mike, all of the tests have revealed that you are a candidate for surgery," he said, explaining that the tests had pinpointed a scar on the right side of the brain. Dr. Waltz felt that through brain surgery, the scar could be removed and I stood a good chance of being seizure free for the rest of my life.

I immediately popped to attention. We were getting somewhere after all. Maybe there was hope, and just maybe I had reason to look ahead to a life where fear was eliminated and the shackles were removed.

My God, I couldn't imagine a life without seizures. Could there be such a thing? I mean, I've never thought there could be such a thing.

It was then that Dr. Waltz looked me straight in the eyes, and calmly said, "But I want you to know there is a risk."

"So, what kind of risk is there?" I queried.

"Well, there's a one to two percent chance of a stroke during surgery," he explained. "I just want you to know that."

I have always been one who worries a lot, but this was one time when I knew I had to make a decision. "That's not much of a risk, considering everything," I quickly said. "One of these things (seizures) is going to kill me before the surgery will anyway. Let's go for it."

Up until that point, I had been brave. I had shunned the illness, trying not to make people be concerned for me. To me, fighting the illness was just part of life. But for the first time, I got scared when Dr. Waltz dropped the question, "Okay, when do you want to have the surgery?"

It was then that I suddenly began to have second thoughts. Talking about the surgery was easy. Now we were getting down to the nitty gritty, and I was scared.

With the year rapidly winding to an end, I immediately began to look for that magic deadline. "How about after the first of the year?" I responded, thinking that I would have a couple of months to get my real courage together.

My wife has this incredible courage, and it was then that she blurted, "No, let's do it right before Christmas. That way, you can stay home with me and the kids."

Bingo. It was a done deal. No chickening out on this deal. Let's just get this over with. I had a few weeks to contemplate what was going to happen, but that "first of the year" idea was out of the question.

This was the big time, the Final Four of my fight. It was run-and-gun time. No taking the air out of the ball this time. Like the Runnin' Rebels that I covered in the 1970s, it was time to go for it. This was definitely a time to separate the boys from the men, and quite frankly, I wasn't sure at all that I was ready for this.

I immediately started thinking about what might happen if I were to have a stroke. Being stuck in a wheelchair for the rest of my life was something that I had never thought much about until we started scheduling the surgery.

I never said anything to my wife, but the truth was that I was frightened to death inside, as we scheduled the "right side lobectomy" with Dr. Waltz's secretary. They were going inside my skull, and now that the chance had finally arrived, I was honestly having second thoughts.

The date was set. I was to arrive at Scripps Hospital on Dec. 5, 1994 for my blood work, and enter the hospital the following morning at 5:30. The decision had been made, and I was on my way. I would later learn that the right temporal lobe would be removed, clearing the way for a whole new life.

The seizures were controlling my life, and I was tired of being sick. When I'd have a seizure, the left side of my body would go numb. Each seizure was stronger than the one before. And I suddenly had something to remind me of how serious the disorder had become.

One day, while making my favorite fried potatoes and hot dogs, I went into a seizure. I didn't fall, but the room began going around in circles. I didn't realize the severity of the seizure, until I pulled my left hand away from the red-hot pan. I had grabbed the pan without realizing it, and because I didn't feel anything, literally clutched it while in the middle of a seizure. I looked down at my hand, which by now had a huge bubble blister on it. I was stunned by the fact that I didn't feel any pain. For the rest of my life, the palm of my left hand will have a scar, reminding me of that ugly day.

However, the scars were much deeper than the one on my hand. The disorder had scarred me emotionally and physically, and I wasn't backing down. Unable to explain each and every seizure, I began to wonder over and over again what to do. Because of the threat of a seizure, I always felt on guard. Until later in my life, I didn't realize that I simply couldn't reach my full potential, because my days were filled with hesitancy and fear. I was continually worrying about what to do in the event of a seizure and truly could not concentrate on one particular challenge or topic. It seems that everything began to go into a fog at that moment. Now that I look back, I can't remember many things that took place between the scheduling of the surgery and the actual procedure.

Our first Thanksgiving in our newly built house would literally be erased from my mind. With the feast only two weeks prior to the surgery, I was apparently so preoccupied with fear that I would eventually discover that the period of my life would only be relived through the reminders given to me by my family. We had a giant gathering with my wife's family at the house for Thanksgiving, but it wasn't until the fall of 1995 that I would be able to remember where we had dinner. Obviously, things were racing through my mind. Nevertheless, I kept telling myself that the surgery I was about to face wasn't any big deal.

This was, however, a lot tougher than I had anticipated. I wasn't letting on, but my emotional state wasn't good. When I told people that I was having brain surgery, the first response was, "Yeah, sure."

As the day I was to enter Scripps neared, I began to feel myself starting to really tighten up. I shared my fear with a few good friends, but tried to keep the situation to myself. I couldn't let down now, not after all the years of suffering. There was no backing down now, even though the first thing that popped into my head each morning was that I was a day closer to brain surgery.

The seizures worsened, possibly because the stress had become more intense than ever before. Truthfully, I began to wonder if I was going to make it to the operating table.

CHAPTER 17
D-DAY IS NEARING

The period between Thanksgiving and my entrance into Scripps Hospital is something I cannot re-create. The memory of that period of my life has been erased for unknown reasons. All I know is that I was desperately attempting to come to grips with the biggest decision of my life.

Everything began to build up on me. While my public relations/ advertising business was beginning to thrive, I was ignoring a huge problem. As I would later discover, I was hiding my fear, failing to discuss my concerns with anyone.

In the long run, we would discover that as a family, we all needed to sit down in a room together and discuss what was about to happen. We were so caught up with building a house and surviving that we had swept under the rug an event in our lives that was more important than any of us knew. For instance, what if something happened during surgery? We had been warned there was a chance, but I shrugged all of that off. People thought I was being brave. I just didn't know any other way to handle what was about to happen.

We had gone from an eighteen hundred and thirty square-foot home to this massive thirty-eight hundred square foot palace. Adjusting to a new home with a house payment four times that of the previous note was tough enough.

It's true that we all tend to take on too many big decisions at once. Our plate wasn't full. It was overflowing, and we didn't even know it.

I kept hesitating when telling my friends about the surgery. I'm a person who had come from a topsy-turvy background, and it seemed that just about the time I got my hopes up, the roof caved in. I kept wondering if the surgery would really help. Surely, nothing else had helped up to this point, so why would I ever be blessed with anything so wonderful as a day without seizures? There was sure to be a glitch, I feared.

The next worry was my insurance. Surely, with the way the insurance was carefully diagnosing everything, we'd be certain to run into a problem with coverage. *The Nifty Nickle* was my employer at the time. The Las Vegas advertisement publication was owned by Cap Cities, which also owned ABC TV and ESPN. I had never tested their insurance, but could just see getting lost in the numbers with another corporate giant.

It was a meeting with *Nifty Nickle* General Manager Bill Davis that helped me open the final door to the surgery. Davis called me into his office, saying he wanted to discuss the surgery with me. "Mike, I want you to listen to me for a minute," Davis said. "You need to make sure that you follow particular steps, so that you'll have the surgery covered. Make sure you get in touch with the insurance company to get the procedure covered."

Carmen had said she didn't care about the insurance. "If they don't cover it, we'll pull the money out of the house. You're going to get well, one way or the other."

But Davis had a good point. Frankly, I hadn't thought about the insurance, choosing instead to leave it in the hands of others. I figured that all I had to do was show up at the door of Scripps Hospital and plop down my insurance card.

It was then that I began making phone calls, and the woman on the other end of the line was someone who, like me, had suffered from chronic illness. In this case, the woman on the other end of the line had multiple sclerosis. She seemed to understand what I had been going through, and immediately began providing me with the necessary information.

To a degree, it was almost like she was cheering me on to get well. "Don't worry, we'll make sure you're taken care of," she assured me. "All we need is the costs of the surgery faxed to us, and we'll go from there."

This was starting to go too smoothly, I thought.

The estimate came back from Dr. Waltz's office in a very short period of time. The surgery and eight-day stay at Scripps Hospital—considered the best in the world by some—came to about twenty-six thousand dollars. I shuddered to think that the insurance company would balk and I'd head back home with more seizures facing me again.

However, I was wrong. The approval came back as fast as it had been faxed from Dr. Waltz, and I had passed another hurdle. What I would later discover was that the cost of the surgery at Scripps was far less than I might have expected in Las Vegas, where medical costs are generally considered some of the highest in the country. In addition to that, the medical profession has been highly questioned in Las Vegas, especially with something as serious as brain surgery.

So, here I was, heading for the best hospital in the world, in the hands of two of the finest doctors in the world. That's not to mention the staff of Scripps, which I would later discover was absolutely invaluable. Scripps Hospital was where Mother Theresa went when she needed help. Now, I was going there. I suddenly began to perk up, and have true hope in this battle. In the back of my mind, though, I questioned if the surgical procedure would work.

Just as a reminder, the seizures continued. And the time of departing was nearing. Needless to say, I was getting a little more scared every day.

Little did I know that I was about to begin a journey that would literally change my whole life.

A racing enthusiast, I was about to leave my life in the pits and head for Victory Circle. They were taking down the yellow flags of my life and pulling out the checkered flag. I was being pushed from the pits, and I had my foot to the throttle. There was a victory at the end of this series of hiccups. I began to pick up stamina, something I had never experienced before.

Get after it, I thought. *Don't give up now.*

I had too many people in my corner, too many teammates on my pit crew.

There was hope and I would find the answer to all of this. I just needed the team, the people to encourage me to win this war.

Race car drivers like Richard Petty never won a race without their pit crew. Golfers count on their caddies for guidance. They have confidence and for good reason. I had my caddies, my pit crew and all the rest. We couldn't lose now.

CHAPTER 18
THE LONGEST DAY OF MY LIFE

We began to scramble to get my life in order, as we prepared for the trip to Scripps. We had soccer games to attend, and a new house to get together.

There were so many responsibilities to handle in such a short period of time, but we all just kept trudging ahead.

On the night before the journey to Scripps, I attempted to lay my head down on the pillow. However, I probably endured the longest night— to be followed by the longest day—of my life. I was excited, but scared at the same time. Things were coming together, but there was certainly reason to be concerned.

I awoke the next morning after tossing and turning all night. I dozed lightly, but might as well have stayed up all night long.

When the sun started to rise, I hopped in the shower. Our new home was only twenty minutes from the airport, but I didn't want to take any chances on this one.

We all climbed in the car, and headed down the road. It didn't take long before I would be reminded why we were taking the trip. About a mile from the house, I began to fall into a bad seizure. We pulled off the road so that I could gain my senses, but this was to begin a horrible day,

Everyone was scared, especially me. The kids and Carmen noticed that I was quickly fading. It was so typical, something you never get used to.

They say that tension plays havoc with seizures. Between my lack of sleep and the stress with the decision to have the surgery, I was about to receive the one-two of seizures.

We boarded the plane, and I again felt myself slipping into another seizure only this time, the seizure was worse than the first one I had experienced earlier in the day.

They weren't grand-mal seizures, but they were close. My head was killing me.

Seizures tend to come in clusters. Just about the time I was recovering from one, I'd get hammered with another. About thirty thousand feet above the desert floor, I had another one and all I could think about was that I wasn't going to make it to Scripps.

We arrived in San Diego, and I was so groggy that I could barely hold my head up. Carmen would again ask me if I was okay, I told her everything was fine. Same script, just a different day. But the truth was that I was sick, real sick. We had two of our three sons with us, as I waddled my way through the airport in San Diego to the rental car agency.

It was Dec. 5, 1994, and I was to have my blood work done at Scripps in final preparation for the surgery. The day was growing longer, when while standing in front of the hospital and I went into my fourth seizure of the day.

Carmen spotted the fact that there was trouble, as we stood in front of the hospital, the sea breeze blowing through my hair. She knew right from the get-go that I was having trouble.

"Are you okay?" Carmen frantically asked me.

It was then that I finally let the fear be known. I was less than twenty-four hours from brain surgery, and with the bandage covering the needle marks from my blood work, I staggered to regain my balance. "Carmen, I can't take this anymore," I responded. "I hope to God this works, because I can't take it anymore. I'm telling you that I can't take anymore of these things."

My wonderful wife has an absolutely uncanny way of putting things in perspective. She has more guts than I do, and doesn't fear anything. She doesn't hesitate, and although I've questioned her many times, I must give her credit for a strong inner soul that gives her strength. And it was then than Carmen told me something that will forever remain in my mind. She put her arms around my neck, and looked me in the eyes. "Just think," she said. "Tomorrow, it'll all be over with. They (the seizures) are taking their last shots at you, because they know it's all over with tomorrow. Just look at it that way."

It all sounded so simple, but I didn't believe a word of it. How in the world could all of this end so abruptly after more than thirty years of torture?

I stood there in front of Scripps Hospital, attempting to regain my senses. This sort of thing happened so many times before, and recovering was something that generally took a couple of minutes, unless that horrid grand mal raised its ugly head.

As usual, I was dazed and scared. But what bothered me most was the fact that the entire family had to come to a stop so that I could recover. Good Lord, I couldn't handle everyone paying so much attention to me.

I had begun to feel like an invalid, but I wasn't doing a very good job of dealing with it. This whole thing wasn't normal and my family certainly couldn't be enjoying it anymore than I was. Fathers don't just fade off into another world. They're supposed to be strong, not someone who is in need of constant attention.

I kept thinking about what Carmen had said, but the reality of her statement wasn't sinking into that thick skull of mine. To me, this was something I was stuck with for the rest of my life.

The truth of the matter was that the experience of the seizure in front of Scripps Hospital would forever live in my mind. You see, Carmen was right. It would be the last seizure I'd ever have. By no means was this whole ordeal over, but I had actually started to recover before the surgery had been done. My life with seizures was about to become one without them. Those horrible seizures were about to fade away and there couldn't have been a better setting than in full view of the ocean. Bury those damned seizures. Drown them out of my life, so deep into the past that I'd never have one again.

In a sense, I was casting off onto a new journey, a new life. Carmen was right. I didn't want to believe it, but I was really about to turn the corner.

I was headed for home, in more ways than one. Like a battered warrior who wouldn't give up, I was fighting back. They couldn't beat me down, although there was certainly more than one occasion when I had thought that the only way out of seizures was death.

Little did I know that I had a whole new life facing me. A life without seizures, something I had never experienced before, was just around the corner.

Victory Circle was in full view. I had my foot on the gas.

Chapter 19
Meeting Up With Willie Nelson

The night before the surgery, we received a call from our oldest son John who had decided that he was leaving Las Vegas to journey to Scripps to be with me for the surgery.

John had intended to stay home and study for finals, but he couldn't take the suspense. We received a call in the hotel room, and while I didn't speak with him, I knew from the conversation that he was scared.

Believe me, I don't think he was as scared as I was. When I put my head down on the pillow, I really didn't want to go to sleep. I was afraid of hearing that alarm going off, knowing that the buzzer would signal the short drive down the road to Scripps.

I wanted so badly to get well, but the next challenge became more frightening as we got closer to it. At 4:30 in the morning, the alarm went off and my head jerked. My stomach hurt, but I headed for the shower. I wasn't about to back down now.

Scripps Hospital is only about two hundred yards south of Torrey Pines Inn, which is situated along a golf course overlooking the Pacific Ocean. But that drive was one that had me watching every inch of the road.

We entered the hospital doors, and I really began to tense up. But Scripps is comprised of class people, and their ability to handle the concerns of others is something that I will never forget.

I walked up to the check-in desk at 5:30 a.m., and the nurses were waiting for me. Everything was in order, and we gathered in the foyer to await a nurse who would explain the procedure.

"You have three things that you will be asked after the surgery," I was told. "They will first ask you your name and where you're at. You will also be asked the President of the United States."

Knowing that I had a horrible memory anyway, our seventeen-year-old son Joe had reminded me, "Dad, just remember when they ask you about the President that you tell them it's the guy who smoked dope."

These were serious times, but Joe was able to keep me loose. And as I would later learn, keeping me loose at a time like this was the most important part of the ordeal.

A short time later, they led me into my hospital room, and the family gathered around. I tried to be brave, but I could see the fear in the eyes of our ten-year-old, Jeffrey.

About the time I got comfortable, a hospital priest would show up and offer me communion. Since I wasn't Catholic, he said I couldn't take communion, but that he would say a prayer for us. The prayer was very soothing and I proceeded to try and keep a strong composure. I was wheeled into the pre-op room, an area for patients preparing for surgery. There must have been five to six people all heading for surgery, so by no means did I feel alone. I was understandably scared, but a kindly nurse whose job was to speak with the patients came to my side.

She was God sent. I looked up at the clock and we were one hour from the 7:30 a.m. trip to the operating room. I kept glancing at the clock, as the seconds continued to tick away. The nurse began to move around the room, asking each person why they were there.

We could all hear what the other was saying, as the nurse spoke softly to each patient. The woman next to me was having a breast removed and I cringed. I was having serious surgery, but felt bad for her. She sounded brave, as I could tell.

I kept my head on the pillow, and for the life of me, I don't know why I did what I did then. For some reason, I looked up to the ceiling and whispered, "Please God, please take care of me."

Mind you, I had never been a spiritual person before, but I had begun experiencing spirituality in the past few weeks. I had never asked God for help, but I needed Him now.

And I will never forget that it was at this point that my arms actually relaxed. There was a relaxed feeling I had never experienced before, and here I was about to have an overhaul on a sputtering message center.

"Honey, what are you having done?" the kindly nurse asked.

"Oh, I'm having a right-side lobectomy," I replied.

"Sounds like you're having seizures," she said.

"Uh yeah, about thirty years' worth. It's been awfully tough," I said.

I don't recall the nurse's name, but her sincere care for my well being is something that I will always remember. She told me of how people with seizures are many times misunderstood. "I remember that we had a busboy in Boston who had them all the time," she said. "It seemed that the only people who understood them were his fellow busboys. Nobody had time to understand him."

Did I ever understand how that fellow must have felt. People don't have time for you when you're sick many times. But the nurse had time for me, and that was nice.

"Everything will be fine for you," she assured me. "You have two of the greatest doctors in the world."

I had faith for the first time in my life. In fact, I was so strong that I didn't even need a pre-op shot to settle me down. For some reason, I was at peace with myself.

"By the way," the nurse said, "you'll get a kick out of the fact that your anaesthesiologist's name is Willie Nelson."

"Oh good," I responded. "Here I am coming from Las Vegas where we have the National Finals Rodeo and I've got a guy named Willie Nelson giving me drugs."

Little did I know that Willie Nelson was another example of the fascinating philosophy of Scripps Hospital. The clock ticked away, and I couldn't wait to meet this guy.

"Hey, what's your name?" I asked when Willie looked down on me.

"Bill Nelson," was the reply.

"You mean, Willie Nelson?" I said.

"That's me, baby,"he said. "I'm the original dirtbag. C'mon with me, cause you're going to surgery."

That trip down the hallway turned into chatter between myself and the guy who will never be forgotten. But when I saw the letters "OR" on the operating room wall, I knew this was the big time.

Willie wasn't done with me yet, as I would soon discover. When he slid me from the gurney to the operating table, I suddenly discovered that sparkling silver tabletop was cold as ice.

"My God, this thing is cold," I told Willie.

"Well, we've got to keep you awake," he replied. "Got to keep things lively."

After adjusting to the cold of the operating table, I looked up at that huge light and began to think about things. Quite frankly, I was hoping Willie would hurry up and give me something to knock me out.

But he wasn't done with me yet, as I would soon discover. I heard him ask the nurse whether the surgery required a general or a local anesthetic. I had known from watching the surgery on television that I was going to be knocked out, since the damage was on the right side of the brain.

The left side of the brain is your speech area, so patients must remain awake during surgery. During the surgery, doctors speak with the patient, making sure not to remove the portion of the brain that controls the speech. If the patient goes mute, they then know to leave that area alone.

"Willie, we're having a general anesthetic," I said, knowing well that I wanted no part of being awake during this thing. "It's a right-side lobectomy."

Willie Nelson had me right where he wanted me. When I responded like I did, he had hooked the big fish and he was going to take his time reeling his catch.

Willie glanced across to a book that was propped next to the surgical table. He began thumbing through the pages. "Hmm, you're right," Willie said with a dead panned look on his face. "It's a right-side lobectomy, all right."

I began to wonder about Willie Nelson, and we were literally minutes from brain surgery. There was no time to head out of this place, though. I could have been the first person in the history of brain surgery to jump off the operating table and high tail his way out of Scripps in a gown.

"Wait a minute!" I said, raising my head from the table. "You mean you could have taken out the wrong side of my brain?"

Willie Nelson was on stage, and he wasn't about to let me off the hook at that point. "Oh well, what the hell," he said. "Worse things have been known to happen, you know."

It didn't take a split second for me to fire back. "Like what?!" I said, literally dumbfounded by what I was hearing.

We were headed for the races and Willie was in high gear. "Well, see that young lady next to you?"

"Uh, yeah," I said, looking at the nurse who was standing by my right side.

"Well, we did surgery on her and it didn't work."

"What in the hell did you do?" I said, beginning to pick up steam just when I was supposed to be mellowing out.

"Well, I'll put it to you like this," Willie said. "She came in a nymphomaniac, and she went out a nymphomaniac."

"Uh, okay."

Willie looked down at me and signaled that the show was about to end.

"Give me your hand because you're going to sleep," he said.

The needle was in my left hand and I didn't have time to count backward from ten. Within two seconds, the room was dark and I was gone.

And Willie Nelson, the showman of the Scripps Hospital Operating Room, will forever live in my mind for his ability to keep things lively. He was actually a fun experience during some very frightening times.

CHAPTER 20

THANK GOD THEY NEVER
WARNED ME....

It has often been said that some things are better left unsaid. And when you're talking about brain surgery that could never have been more certain.

While I was aware that a small portion of damaged brain matter would be removed during surgery, I had never really given the procedure much thought. In other words, I never really delved into what was going to take place after Willie Nelson put me to sleep.

Quite frankly, I'm glad I never became too inquisitive about the process, because I'm afraid that I would have chickened out before Willie almost sent me beating feet for Black's Beach.

In order to prepare the scalp, my head was shaved on the ride side. From there, a cut was made from above the temple above the right eye. The incision went down the side of my head behind the right ear and curled just behind the ear lobe. As I would later discover, the scalp was pulled forward to reveal the skull. Knowing exactly where they needed to open the skull, doctors Waltz and Aung then used saws and drills to cut a piece of the skull just above the right ear.

While it has never been proven, I'm sure Aung and Waltz may have considered a jackhammer for the procedure, considering the fact that I have been accused of having the hardest skull ever. They undoubtedly earned their money when it came time to work on me.

This was nothing less than an "ugly" procedure. The skull apparently burns, and water is needed to cool the friction, which is created by the cuts that are made. The skull is unforgiving, especially when one considers that it is mine, and it takes aggressiveness to open it to get to the brain.

Hell, if miners had to get through something as tough as my skull, the gold rush would never have taken place. They would have thrown down their picks and shovels and gone off to do something else. Your head literally becomes somewhat of a cookie jar in brain surgery. The area is opened, and in my case, five centimeters of brain matter were removed, just about the limit that can be taken without taking too many chances. I had two of the best doctors in the world and I was in good hands.

I would later remind my kids not to make fun of my absent-mindedness, considering that I only had part of my brain. In fact, I'd milk that one as much as I could. I thought back to a conversation that I had once with Dr. Aung, who told me he always wanted to see the Imperial Palace Auto Collection. Like me, he loved relic cars. A good friend of mine named Denny Selleck once had open-heart surgery. When he interviewed his doctor, he made his selection based on the fact that the surgeon loved to tinker with automobiles. Denny felt that if the doctor could rebuild a motor, he could rebuild his heart. Just the mere fact that Dr. Aung loved cars gave me a sense of comfort. I never asked Dr. Waltz if he liked cars, but figured one of the two was good enough for me.

So, my two "mechanics" went to work on my brain, and began reworking the wiring system that had been damaged by so many short-circuits. They knew exactly where they were going, and took three and a half hours to put my life together.

It seemed that I awoke almost as fast as I had gone to sleep. Understandably, I was dizzy when I woke up. I was somewhat confused. But more than anything else, I had the worst headache of my life. The saws and drills had gotten through my head, but not without leaving me in excruciating pain.

"Mr. Henle, are you okay?" a nurse asked.

I seem to remember her asking me if I could hear all right. I struggled to find my senses. I had never been in such pain before. Middle-of-the-night seizures hadn't been this bad.

"Uh, I think I'm okay," I responded. "But my head hurts so bad. Can you give me something for the pain?"

The nurse informed me I had already received a shot. Another was on its way. I was being introduced to morphine. All I knew was that one dose of it wasn't enough. Somebody had better get hold of Willie Nelson, because his drugs worked better.

A tube had been inserted in the side of my head to alleviate the pressure, so I was lying on my back with my head turned to the left. It was about then that I would encounter a very real experience long before Della Reese had made *Touched By An Angel* a television hit. As I looked to my left, I saw the face of my mother-in-law, who had passed away of cancer about eight months earlier. Arline Rivero had been like a mother to me, and her loss was something that hurt all of us. Upon seeing her, I attempted to make sense of what was happening. I blinked my eyes, as I looked to my left. Arline was just sitting there looking ahead. She always looked out for us, and seemed to be looking out for me. She was a woman of few words, but her mere presence had always been a wonderful part of our lives.

I didn't want to say anything to anyone about seeing Arline. I had wondered if something had gone wrong during surgery. But she was there, just sitting up to my left in somewhat of a cloud. Long-time friend Bill Morris would later explain that Arline Rivero was my guardian angel during some very dangerous times. Once he explained it to me, it all made sense. A short time later, the popularity of angels hit an all-time high.

The nurse began asking more questions, the same ones that I had been told would be asked of me after the surgery. "We'd like to ask you a few questions," she said. "First, what is your name?"

I answered that one okay.

"Where are you now?"

Scripps Hospital. Hell, this was easy.

"Do you know who is the president of the United States?"

Bingo. Remember, Joe told me to remember that it's the guy who smoked dope. "Bill Clinton," I responded.

"Now, I'd like you to squeeze my fingers as hard as you can," the nurse instructed.

I reached over and squeezed her hand. There, everything seemed to work. I could even still type. I could relax a little more. Everything seemed to work. I survived this far, and other than the headache, I wasn't doing too badly. My pit crew was doing its job and I was on my way. The epilepsy was getting the black flag. I was getting the green flag. It wasn't long before I'd get to Victory Circle.

CHAPTER 21

THE GREATEST PIT CREW ON EARTH

The headache finally began to subside, and it was time to be taken back to my room. Dr. Aung met with my family and informed them he and Dr. Waltz had taken longer than expected, just to make certain all of the scar tissue had been removed from the brain.

After a while in the "step down room" (otherwise known as "Recovery" in most hospitals), it was time to head for my room to see my family.

I kept dozing and finally woke up to see Carmen and the kids in my room. Things were understandably foggy, but other than the tube hanging out the side of my head like an overflow line from a radiator, I knew that everything was about as normal as could be expected.

I vaguely remember the boys and Carmen asking me if I was okay. It was so good to hear their voices, although I couldn't respond much. Before long, the phone began to ring, as friends and family called to see how I was doing.

As luck would have it, one of my recovery nurses was an auto race fan. We instantly hit if off and I began babbling about auto racing before the post-surgery medicine could wear off.

Crystal was the nurse's name and her husband was an auto racer. Hell, there was no surgery that could keep me from talking about the run for the checkered flag and I was discussing motor sports while I probably should have been sleeping.

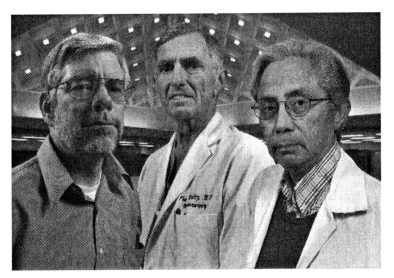

Ten years after the surgery, I joined two of my greatest friends neurosurgeon Dr. Thomas Waltz, center; and neurologist Dr. M.H. "Andy" Aung.

That god-awful tube, complete with its pouch that was to collect the fluid from the brain, was the focus of my first concerns after I had returned to my room. Carmen began to notice that the bag on my right shoulder was filling quickly with blood. When she asked Crystal about the situation, I began to panic. I didn't say anything to anyone, but privately I began asking myself if we had made a mistake by having the surgery done.

As groggy as I was, I remember a call for Dr. Waltz. The bag was beginning to fill. *My God*, I thought. *Don't tell me we've got to go back for this again.*

Dr. Waltz arrived a short time later. He was calm, and his voice quickly erased my fears. He tells you up-front what you're facing, but he doesn't express fear. I guess the one thing I learned out of all the years of seizures was that panic showed by others tends to complicate matters.

It's just incredible how much a soothing voice can help calm a frightened person. Dr. Waltz had an incredible mannerism about him. When he walked into the room, there was a sense of peace that seemed to radiate itself. I would be okay, and I could tell that by the way he handled the situation.

The nurses smiled and the doctors were confident. Good Lord, I couldn't have been in better hands. The tube was a drag, but had to make for good photos.

Life had been so chaotic before, so topsy-turvy. And here was a man and his team that wasn't concerned outwardly about the post-operative results.

It was determined that my upper body was simply elevated too much and Dr. Waltz made the adjustment. It was no big deal. We just changed the suspension on the bed and readied me for the rest of the race.

I had figured out that Dr. Thomas Waltz could have been the ideal crew chief for an auto racing team. Race teams need people who can remain calm during tense times. Both Dr. Waltz and Dr. Aung— along with all of the people of Scripps—were there to resurrect my life.

I had just survived life-threatening surgery and the team at Scripps was so calm. I arrived in the room and they became like an extended family. From the nurses to the doctors and the janitors, I felt like everyone was there to cheer me on.

I was in a hospital room and felt like I was standing in front of one hundred thousand fans giving me a standing ovation. We weren't done with this battle yet, but the motor was fresh and we were running on all eight cylinders.

This command center of mine had been reworked and we were just going through a bit of a "shakedown." If there was any kind of problem, I was certain my pit crew would simply repair the problem and we'd move on. At Scripps, there was a security blanket that I had never experienced before. Everyone handled situations so well. They met brain surgery with confidence, and even though there was

MIKE HENLE

a chance of seizures after the surgery, I felt that there were people there to immediately offer psychological and moral help.

For five grand-mal seizures and literally thousands of petit-mal seizures, I had tried to hide. It was much easier just to disguise my fear and go on with my life. But the seizures had become too much to hide and my search for a miracle was about to become successful.

Dr. Waltz and Dr. Aung were removing a very ragged part of my life. I was about to find out how wonderful life could be without seizures.

78

CHAPTER 22
THE ONE FACE I DIDN'T WANT TO SEE

The one thing I noticed immediately about Scripps was the positive people. There wasn't anyone who had a negative philosophy on life. If it wasn't the calm voices, it was the smile on everyone's face. It appeared that the set for the movie *Patch Adams* had been established long before the script had even been written. Robin Williams would love this place. It was proof that good health and success in life has a direct relationship to good attitudes. When you're around the people of Scripps, it's easy to maintain a good attitude, no matter who you're speaking with.

A day after the surgery, I was wheeled downstairs for another EEG to monitor the surgery and check on any possible seizure patterns. I innocently glanced around the room, noticing that others were heading for the same procedure as I was.

Upon being wheeled into the room, one of the nurses commented that she and the staff had seen the surgery via television the day before. I found that fascinating, thinking that I was the center of attention on the Scripps television system. Hell, I was somewhat of a celebrity.

"You did very well," she said. "It was very aggressive surgery, but you did well."

After about an hour of having wires pasted to my skull, I was wheeled back into the waiting area. I had been through this procedure so many times that I almost could have wired myself to the machine.

On one hand, I didn't want to see the results of the test. But on the other, there was a sense of confidence in knowing that everything would be okay.

I looked around and without thinking, glanced right at a man who had told me sometime earlier that the surgery was too dangerous. There, in full view, was Dr. Jack Sipe standing about ten to fifteen feet from me. I instantly noticed that my right eye was swollen. Sipe's original fear that the surgery was too close to the optic nerve suddenly became a concern. The sight of Sipe was almost like a television close-up. I instantly wanted to change the channel.

For the first time, I noticed that I had double vision. And suddenly, I had a fear that Jack Sipe would wander over to my gurney and inform me that I had made a serious mistake. I looked up to the ceiling and hoped that Sipe would either not recognize me or simply ignore the fact that I was there.

If there were any negative people at Scripps, I was certain it was Sipe. And one day after surgery, I ran right into him. The timing couldn't have been worse.

I was taken into the room for the EEG, wired up and put through the test. In my mind was the concern that everything would be okay.

When the test was concluded, the nurses wheeled me back into the waiting area to be taken back to my room. I couldn't wait to see Dr. Aung again. A short time after arriving back in my room, Dr. Aung strolled in with a smile on his face. "We have very good news," he said. "We got all of the damaged matter. You're going to be fine."

"That's wonderful news, Dr. Aung," I responded. "However, I have one question. We didn't hurt the optic nerve, did we?

"No, we were very careful with that," Dr. Aung responded. "Dr. Waltz pulled it aside during surgery and showed me. He was very careful about that. Everything is going to be fine."

"I was concerned, because I'm having a little problem with my eyesight," I said. "I was just concerned that something may be wrong."

Dr. Aung reassured me that the double vision was simply the result of tofus or swelling of the area near the surgery. Since the right eye was so close to the beginning of the cut, there was a natural tendency to swell.

"Good," I said. "I saw Jack Sipe down in the EEG area and it worried me because he was afraid of the surgery. Do me one big favor, would you? Go down and tell him we kicked his butt!"

Dr. Aung smiled, displaying that look of confidence. Whereas I'm the type of person who celebrates by shouting to the mountains, Dr. Aung was so mellow. I could tell that he, too, felt good about our "victory," although his way of celebrating was much different than my own.

I felt like the football player who had just run one hundred yards for a touchdown. If we had been on the football field, I would have spiked the ball into the ground or thrown it into the stands and done a little dance.

If I had just won the Indy 500, I would have taken a swig of milk.

To me, Dr. Aung had just waved the checkered flag or signaled a touchdown. That's all that mattered. We all had faith and I was reaching for the sky.

I closed my eyes and thanked God. We were still winning this fight—and Victory Circle was just around the corner.

CHAPTER 23
TAKING ONE STEP AT A TIME

The stitches hadn't healed yet, and I was already beginning to get around a few days after the surgery. The nurses would wake me up in the middle of the night to give me the various assortment of post-operative medication and as much as I hated taking the medicine, their pleasant demeanor was something that I looked forward to.

The days to go home were drawing closer, and there was a sense of sadness on my part. Doctors carefully monitored me throughout the day and I had never felt so protected.

I wasn't fond of the steroids needed to keep the swelling of the brain down and I never have liked pain medicine. But best of all, I still was free of seizure activity. There wasn't even a sign of a petit-mal seizure and I was feeling better every day. I'd climb out of bed and walk around the hallways, steering the small contraption that had the bag for intravenous feeding.

I had to be one of the most interesting sights in the hospital, with my head shaved and the tube sticking out the side. It had to resemble Cyclops with the horn sticking out of the side rather than the center of my head, but I was in good spirits.

The entire experience was actually somewhat interesting. Every day, I'd meet someone else new and thank my lucky stars for such wonderful people. I've always been one who could strike up a conversation with everyone and it was no different in a hospital.

One nurse in particular, a young girl named Julie, came in daily to give me my medicine and shoot the breeze. She was a fan of the Grateful Dead, and I'd greet her with, "Hey, it's the dead head!"

When Julie wasn't on day shift, she was the nurse who woke me up in the middle of the night. She was always a welcomed sight, because she had such an interesting outlook on life. "Just remember not to panic, no matter what happens," said Julie one day when I asked her about the possibility of having another seizure. "I always remember never to panic, especially when scuba diving or sky diving."

That phrase stuck in my mind. I had generally been a person who worried about everything, and those soothing words worked better than any sedative I had ever taken.

Ironically, it was Julie's words that came to mind when, while taking my medicine, I began to choke. In the past, choking many times accompanied seizures. There was no seizure this time, but I could tell that the pills and the water had gone down the wrong pipe. I then thought about Julie's advice and rather than throw my arms up in the air, I just calmed down. The pills slid down my throat and I went on with my life. It was so easy, and the end result was certainly better.

Piece of cake, I thought. Just listen to your nurses and everything will be fine.

Doctors had determined that I was doing well after about five days and plans were under way to send me home after eight days. Each day became a little more enjoyable and I seemed to be moving about a little better. I continued to hang around the nurses' stand during my walks, leading my little contraption with me like a race crew member does a toolbox. I had actually become accustomed to the damned thing.

My God, I thought to myself. *I'm really not sick at all anymore.* As long as everyone was around me, I was doing pretty well. I was actually getting used to the radiator hose sticking out the side of my head. Everything was going well, I thought, and the pace of the hospital was so nice and slow.

There was no rushing around or drag racing from one place to another. I was in hog heaven, actually learning a new way of life with a brand new brain.

My folks called right after the surgery and so did my godfather, a farmer named Cliff Kramer from a little ranch near Knights Landing.

It felt good knowing that people cared enough to call.

The calls had to be driving the girls on the switchboard nuts. It seemed that half the world was calling, and that was good for my mental state. Carmen and the kids had gone home a few days after the surgery and while the folks of Scripps were very helpful, I badly needed interaction with family members and friends.

At this time, I began to really concentrate on home—not Las Vegas, but Northern California. I began to long for the view of green fields and rivers. I had begun going back to my youth for some reason, thinking back about the years past. In my time to relax, I just kind of mulled over the past, charting my route.

As time went by, I felt so comfortable at Scripps. It had become so much a part of my life and I had become used to the hospital and its staff. I'd walk around until I found a window with a view of the ocean and just think about things. There was no better place to recover than Scripps Hospital and its proximity to the ocean.

Just when I had really gotten used to the tube, one of the nurses mentioned that it was about time to take it out. I certainly didn't want to go home with the hose hanging out of the side of my head.

No big deal, I thought. *What the hell, it couldn't be that big of a deal pulling it out of the skull.*

And was I ever wrong. I suddenly had to think back about what Julie had told me. Just relax and don't panic. The attendant said there would be slight dull pain when he began to pull the tube out. He placed his hand squarely on the center of my back, and I waited.

And when the tube began coming out, there was this horrible dull ache inside the skull cavity. The entire right side of my head hurt badly. In fact, it kind of felt like there was a suction, and I began to wonder if there was any brain matter going to be left by the time they pulled the radiator hose out of the side of my head.

The hospital personnel would later tell us that all that was left were the staples that needed to be removed from the side of my head. While I never inquired how many there were, there had to be dozens. I must have looked like Frankenstein.

Removing the staples was not painful, nothing like when the hose was pulled out of the side of my head. The nurses had said we could wait until we got home to remove them, but after some discussion, it was determined that we could "unzip" my head while at Scripps. The nurse grabbed what appeared to be a pair of pliers and began removing the staples one by one. There was no pain and it didn't feel like anything was falling out. I looked down to my right side and didn't see anything alongside the bed, so I knew the staple job had to work well.

The bionic man was holding together and the seizures were staying away. What else could a guy like me ask for?

I began thinking of what all of us had been through. My whole life was actually one war after another because of the seizure disorder. Now, we had all gathered like warriors battling the enemy. And the most important thing of all was that we were winning. The enemy— epilepsy—was retreating and we were getting ready to raise the flag.

The people of Scripps had become more than just hospital personnel. They had become part of my family, members of a platoon that blind-sided the enemy and sent him packing.

I had been saved by the people of Scripps Hospital, who had taken a badly beaten and wounded man and put him together for the first time in his life. They all seemed to take for granted what they had done for me, but I was like a little kid who had opened his eyes for the first time ever.

We were winning this war and it was about time to pack up our gear and head home. I began to understand what soldiers felt like after a big battle had been won. I was about to leave my comrades of Scripps, and honestly felt somewhat sad about my departure. In a sense, I kind of resembled a wounded but happy and victorious soldier. I had been a prisoner of war for so long and now it was time to return to my homeland. Until now, I had been held captive by epilepsy. The people of Scripps had unlocked the handcuffs that the disorder had produced.

By no means were we done. Recovery would require patience, but the journey home was about to begin.

Chapter 24
It's Time to Go Home

While the entire staff of Scripps Hospital had become like very close friends, one talented individual really gained a place in our hearts for her dedication and huge smile that she carried into the room every day.

Kate Culliton had been with us from the outset and it was only fitting that a farewell meeting with her take place as we prepared to leave Scripps. For those who must endure an ordeal like brain surgery, a person like Kate Culliton is invaluable. A clinician, she knew how serious the surgery had been, yet Kate tackled the procedure with an uncanny personality that kept all of us alive with new energy.

Kate Culliton was there during the surgery and she was side-by-side with the doctors when I was taken back to my room. When we did not fully understand the surgery or the terms that went along with it, Kate opened the doors for us with an explanation.

When I first came to Scripps to research the idea of surgery, it was John Polich, Ph.D., an associate member of the department of neuropharmacology, who would greet me. He would proceed to inform me that the winning team of Dr. Thomas Waltz and Dr. Maung "Andy" Aung were the best in the world. I'd never forget his words as we rode down from one part of Scripps to the other in his sports car.

And while John Polich lived in my mind for our first days at Scripps in 1994, it would be Kate Culliton that I would remember most for her undying efforts to keep everyone together during the nitty-gritty of surgery and follow-up.

It was Dec. 13, 1994 and my bags were packed. Kate bounced into the room, her smile radiating warmth into the room. When she walked into a room, the whole place came alive, no matter how serious the situation.

Carmen arrived at the hospital, just in time to see the nurse remove the staples. There was still an indentation in the skull, and the hair was closely cut. The right eye was swollen slightly but other than that, I was ready to go.

And most importantly, there had been no seizures since the day before the surgery.

"You need to remember some things," Kate would tell me before we left. "First, you need to understand that seizures are still a possibility. But don't freak out if you have one. You're still in that period when it could happen, but don't worry about it. Second, be sure to get three square meals a day. And remember that you must continue taking your meds (medications). And finally, remember that you're prone to depression. You've been through very serious surgery and you need to be aware of that."

The final statement really didn't sink into my head, although it certainly should have. Depression was a huge concern, although I didn't want to believe it. Kate had never been wrong about anything before, and her words this time certainly carried weight.

Kate and the team of Scripps doctors wished me a farewell, told us that they were just a phone call away and urged us not to worry. But there was something very frightening about leaving Scripps for Las Vegas. I was taken by wheelchair to the car and waved goodbye to everyone.

Las Vegas had been very good to me, but not having the people of Scripps within a few feet bothered me. It wasn't like we could hop in the car and find help for complications from brain surgery. Hopefully, all would go well and we'd move on with our lives.

We had received several medications, including the steroids to keep the swelling of the brain in check. Everything was placed in one bag, Kate wished us well and Carmen was given an inventory list of the medications.

We headed for the beach in San Diego just for last-hurrah looks. I looked at the ocean and didn't say anything, but I was truly frightened. It was so beautiful in San Diego and I was about to lose my security blanket.

A few hours later, we'd climb aboard a Southwest Airlines flight for Las Vegas. I began idle chatter with the stewardess, and suddenly found that she, too, had undergone brain surgery because of injuries suffered in an auto accident.

I began drinking a 7-Up and eating peanuts, talking up a storm. Nobody could imagine that I had been lying on an operating table only eight days before. I was hardly like someone who had been through such an ordeal.

The forty-minute flight went quickly, since I was having the time of my life with the people on the airplane. It was Christmas time, and I was heading back to a brand new home during a festive season.

The boys met us at the airport, and wheeled me to the baggage area, where I encountered a horrible nightmare. I instantly knew that I should have stayed at Scripps.

"Mike, where is your medicine?" Carmen asked.

Confused and frightened, I mumbled and asked if she didn't have it. I searched the seat of the wheelchair and couldn't find my medicine.

My God, I'm going to die. Here I was in Las Vegas three hundred miles from Scripps Hospital and the medicine was gone. The airport was a buzz of activity and there wasn't a soul who could help us. We were all terrified, and I began wondering what in hell we were going to do now. Here it was, nine at night, and I was without the medicine. It wasn't as though we could hop over to the phone and re-order it. I needed it on my first night home for sleep, pain, and seizure control.

I was terrified, as our oldest son Johnny screamed back to the gate of the Southwest flight. A very good athlete, he ran through the airport like a gazelle. Surely, he'd get back to the plane and find the medicine sitting on the seat we had on the way home.

As we would later learn, Johnny vividly recalled the time when at the age of two and a half, I had the grand mal at Dairy Queen. He'd tell us one evening that he remembered the episode, even though he had been so little at the time. With the latest happening at the airport, he had become a part of two very delicate moments in my life and had been there to oversee his dad in both cases. The latest chapter would work itself out, I was sure. However, my world came caving in on me a short time later when Johnny would return to the baggage area— without the medicine.

I had apparently thrown the bag in the garbage without thinking. Dear God, we were in real trouble, I thought. There couldn't possibly have been a more dramatic script written for a movie. All I could do was sit in the wheelchair and cry. I had never been so scared. Good Lord, all of this pain and agony would be for naught if I were to have another seizure now. And the swelling of the brain really concerned me, especially being so far from Scripps.

Carmen retrieved the car and the kids wheeled me to the curb. We scurried home as I lay in the back of the vehicle. I was terrified of the outcome. Our new home was about fifteen minutes from the airport, and we had to be running at Mach I through the streets of southwest Las Vegas.

Luckily, Carmen had kept the inventory sheet in her purse. She called Scripps immediately, and they assured us everything would be okay. We just needed to call our family doctor and have him call the pharmacy for us. It was drag race Las Vegas at its best.

A call to Save On Pharmacy resulted in the nicest pharmacist on earth, who assured us he'd stay open until Carmen could jet to their store to refill the prescriptions.

I went upstairs and climbed into bed. About forty-five minutes later, I heard Carmen screaming into the cul de sac and into the garage. A few seconds later, you could hear the pitter-patter of her running steps coming up the stairway.

I had already climbed into bed, but I was shaking badly. I had never felt so helpless before. Carmen arrived shortly to my bedside, complete with the medication and a glass of water.

And there was one good thing about the near disaster. I didn't have a seizure and generally one accompanied tense moments. There could not have been anything more tense than arriving in the airport without the medication.

I was not only alive, but also seizure-free. It had been a rocky ride back into Las Vegas, but we had survived the landing. I was about to experience my first night home with my "new"brain, which had undoubtedly survived a major test right off the bat.

Chapter 25

It's Not Quite Time to Celebrate

It was wonderful to finally be home after a little "bump in the road." While I had always hated taking medications, this was one time when the sight of the pills was the hand I needed to get back on my feet. Surely, I'd get a good night's sleep and get on with this. I really didn't know whether the medication was going to help, but sure as hell didn't want to take a chance of going without it.

In a brand new house with that brand new brain, I was looking forward to my new life. As strange as it may all sound now, I really didn't know what to expect. Seizures had become so much a part of my life that a life without them was actually something that I could not fathom. It was strange, but interesting. I had always wondered why others were able to deal with matters so much more calmly than I could. Most certainly, a life without seizures could make a big difference in normal everyday functions. Maybe now I could pass my real estate exam, something I had failed on three occasions.

I went out in front of the house and mounted the address. That in itself seemed like something I could never have accomplished before. I had been such a klutz putting things together.

Many of our friends began coming to the house to check on my status. My good friend and neighbor Rod Soesbe was one of the first ones to the house. Many others followed, with a list that included Carmel Hopkins of the *Las Vegas Review-Journal*, homebuilding executive Sue Camara, photographer Tony Scodwell and scads of family members. It was so nice seeing all of our friends. I felt good, almost too good, and began jumping into the workload again before the hair had fully grown back on the side of my head. It was like a coming home party, and I loved seeing the people. Everything seemed to be going so well and the phone began to ring with consistency, as people began calling the house for help with their public relations.

Kate Culliton, my clinician at Scripps, had warned me to take it easy when I got home. She said that full recovery usually took two years. But I felt so good inside and honestly didn't feel as though I had just endured something as serious as brain surgery. In fact, I felt so good that I honestly began not worrying any longer about seizures. Slowly but surely, I was beginning to quit thinking about when the next seizure would riddle my life and cause everyone to come running to my side.

This was really neat, I thought, as my recovery seemed to continue. Surely, I could start putting the pedal to the metal in the drag race world of Las Vegas, where I had thrived as a street-hustling PR guy who literally wore out laptop computers. To me, recovery was based on my interaction with people. What better way than to interact with people and make money at the same time? Hell, I was on a roll again, I said to myself. And besides, I hated to tell people (including the *New York Times*) that I couldn't help them now because of all things, I had just had brain surgery. Kate Culliton's warning wasn't finding its place in that thick skull of mine. I couldn't turn down the chance to work and besides, we had so many things to complete on the house.

I decided to get out of the house with Carmen and accompany her to the grocery store. The damnedest thing struck me, as I entered Smith's Food King. The people were moving so fast, I noticed. My God, this is really rather scary. Everyone is Shirley "Cha Cha" Muldowney and life suddenly seemed like a big whirl. As much as I loved being home, the pace was something that did concern me. I knew inside that Kate had told me to slow down, but it seemed that it was hard to maintain a slow pace when everyone around me was red-lining their tachometer.

I truly wanted to maintain the pace I had adapted at Scripps. It took me a while to slow down, but once I lowered the RPM in my motor, I kind of enjoyed the more methodical lifestyle. I didn't say anything to anyone, but I was truly beginning to become confused. And for the life of me, I was starting to become frightened of things.

Possibly the biggest evidence of that was after awakening one morning a few days after getting home from Scripps, I opened my eyes to the terror that I may have had a seizure in the middle of the night. I wasn't certain, but there was a strange feeling about things. I came downstairs for breakfast and couldn't hold my emotions. I sat at the kitchen table, put my head in my hands, and cried like a baby. Carmen and the kids were sitting at the table, and I struggled to explain to them why I was in tears. I felt so embarrassed by the whole thing and certainly didn't feel like someone who was recovering from my surgery.

I shuddered to think that I had taken a step backwards. On one hand, I wanted to just keep my mouth shut like all the other times I had a seizure. I didn't want anyone worrying about me, and was embarrassed that as a grown man, they had to witness my bawling my eyes out in front of them.

My God, I was forty-four years old. The whole thing seemed so ludicrous.

Carmen quickly called Scripps and all I could think about was that something had gone wrong. Had I just remembered the words of Kate Culliton—another seizure was possible, and not to freak out—I would have been much better off. The friendly physician at Scripps calmly explained to Carmen that I was going to be fine. And in fact, I probably didn't have a seizure anyway. He explained that the brain was so "programmed to having seizures" that it probably didn't even have one. And if a seizure had started, it wasn't possible for it to continue anyway. Only this time, the work of Dr. Aung and Dr. Waltz cut short the seizure. The area of the brain that facilitated the seizures in the past was gone, so there was nothing to worry about. In the meantime, this poor old brain simply like me—had to get used to a life without seizures. In fact, if anything, I probably only had a nightmare that I had had a seizure.

It all made so much sense. I ran upstairs, breathed a sigh of relief and began trudging back into this recovery period. The engine may have sputtered, but it didn't blow. We may have had a little vapor lock, but the motor was running pretty good on all eight cylinders. The key was to give this engine of mine time to break itself in. Hammering the clutch wasn't the thing to do at this point.

Keep thinking about Kate Culliton's words. And don't pull into the front straightaway at one hundred and seventy mph because you're not ready for the action yet. Please, take it easy. Take it slow. Don't be like Elvis and go, man, go.

CHAPTER 26
YET ANOTHER HURDLE

While I continued to physically get better a couple of weeks after arriving home from Scripps, it suddenly occurred to me without forethought that I was about to face another hurdle in my life.

When my clinician Kate Culliton advised me how best to handle the recovery, I really attempted to ignore the idea that I could possibly be a candidate for depression.

My mother had fought depression for countless years, and I was certain that I was too strong to let that sort of thing happen to me. When I left the little town of Yuba City, California, in 1966, I left all of those problems behind me, I thought.

But the fact is that when I returned home from Scripps, depression didn't just come tapping on the door. As I would discover, when depression wants into your life, it can go through the door without turning the handle. The absolute worst thing a person can do is deny the problem, because it is then that depression will take you to the ground.

In my case, I had allowed myself to become a sitting duck. I was a one hundred and fifty-pound linebacker about to be steamrolled by a high-speed, two hundred and forty-five-pound fullback, who had gotten up a massive rush before putting its head and shoulders down to run over me.

The first days back from Scripps were unlike Las Vegas, since rainstorms pelted us. The roof of our home is very steep with no rain gutters and the water came pouring off in buckets. As I lay in bed, the dark gray clouds and the rain were depressing enough.

In Las Vegas, where the earth is hard as a rock, the water runs freely. Washes were wall-to-wall and getting home was next to impossible. The flow of water was controlling the city. Depression was doing the same, running at will over me. It was like a flash flood of emotions and I was quickly losing control.

The wind blew hard, and I shuddered to hear it. I would awake in the middle of the night fearing the sound of the wind and the rain.

Nothing made sense. It never does, when depression begins digging in. Simple addition in the checkbook became unbearable, and writing a one-page press release—something I normally did without a second though— was unbelievably hard.

The *New York Times* called for another front-page story about real estate, and I knew that was out of the question. When I told them what had happened, the editor immediately expressed his concern and offered a get-well.

Losing a chance to write my fifth front-page story for the *New York Times* was very painful. It generally would take weeks to complete and only paid three hundred dollars, but the self-satisfaction of having my by-line in four million papers all over the world produced a feeling that I could never describe.

I was going backwards, and didn't know why. Not being able to run the one hundred-yard dash in ten-flat was something a person could understand, but being frightened of the wind and rain—not to mention my inability to write—was something that I could not figure out.

Surely, I'd arise the next day and everything would be fine. This will surely go away by itself, and I'd just carry on with my life.

However, I was quickly running out of gas, possibly because I was moving too quickly after such serious surgery. A short time after returning home, I had wanted to go to the *Las Vegas Review-Journal* and see some friends.

Halfway to the paper, I had to pull off the road. There weren't any problems with a seizure, but I was literally out of gas. I laid my head down and took a few minutes to regain my senses. It all seemed so silly, but the fact was that I was pushing myself way too much. But I looked so good on the outside. Inside, I was coming apart and didn't even know it.

I finally made it to the *R-J,* where I immediately stopped by to see Carmel Hopkins, a long-time friend, who had taken over my job as real estate editor. One look at me in the doorway and she was stunned. "What in the hell are you doing here?" she quickly asked.

"Uh, well, I just came by to see you," I responded.

"Mike, you just had brain surgery, for Christ sakes! Take this chair and sit down right now."

Everyone could see what I was doing to myself except me. Finally, a good friend and homebuilding executive named Sue Camara told me, "Mike, please get some help."

As the days would drag on, I suddenly became very lonely. A very independent person in the past, I suddenly needed constant attention. I was worse than a little kid.

I had fought the idea that depression could become an overwhelming problem, and didn't want to seek help. I just kept telling myself that I'd get over this fatigue, and life would go on.

I made an appointment to see Mary Keiser, a long-time friend and clinical psychologist. I wasn't fond of seeing a psychologist anyway, but at least Mary was someone that I knew. I trusted her and felt at ease with her, and agreed to meet with her.

Carmen would accompany me to the appointments, and Mary immediately pinpointed a problem. There had been a chemical imbalance, she decided, and the drug Elavil was ordered from Scripps to get things back in order again.

When I discovered that my former editor Carmel Hopkins also took Elavil, I didn't feel like the Lone Ranger. I just hated another crutch, but hearing that someone else took daily doses of the drug was a help.

I immediately began sleeping like never before with the Elavil. With the Elavil and phenobarbital, I began sleeping hard, but it seemed to take forever to wake up. I continued taking both drugs, and everything seemed to be falling together again.

If there had been a chemical imbalance, the Elavil seemed to be eliminating the problem. Other than the fact that I began to put on weight, I was honestly feeling better.

In a telephone conversation with one friend, I would later say that the bout with depression was the toughest battle of my life.

I was so thankful that this war was seemingly over.

Chapter 27

Healing – Physically, Emotionally and Spiritually

In my continued journey to piece everything together, I found myself wandering into St. Joseph's Husband of Mary Catholic Church one day. I had stopped in a shopping center only minutes earlier, and decided to drive up to the church.

I wasn't Catholic, but we had been married in the church more than twenty-three years earlier. I truthfully didn't know the difference between one church and the other, but had found myself wanting to worship.

So, on a gorgeous Saturday afternoon, I pulled into the parking lot and walked to the front of the church. There in front was Father Joseph Anthony. "Young man, can I help you?" he asked, as I looked over the sermon schedules on the window.

"Uh, well, I kind of wanted to see when services were," I responded.

From there, Father Joe asked me if I'd like to speak with anyone at the church about the services offered. He informed me that Deacon Mike Heidenrich was inside the church, and I agreed to have a sit-down chat.

Deacon Mike asked me why I had determined that I should go to church. I told him my story, explaining that I was healthy after so many years of ill health. I explained that I had been given good health, and that was something that I had never experienced before.

I explained that I was very thankful for what I had now, and that going to church was something that seemed important to me, although it had never played a factor in my life before.

"You know, there is a reason why you're here," said Deacon Mike.

I really didn't know what to expect, although I was intrigued by what he said. "You see, we have a young girl who attends church here, and she has epilepsy," he said. "She's really having a tough time. I believe she takes a drug called Dilantin, and her gums are badly swollen. Would you mind coming to speak with her about the disease? I think it would really help her."

I had goose bumps on my arms speaking with Deacon Mike. My God, if there was someone who needed to speak out about his or her problems associated with epilepsy, please lead the way.

As I would later discover, going to church offered such a sense of peace. It was the ideal way to unwind and just think about things. I loved going, although I really didn't understand religion.

I became a member of the church after several months of classes, and was fascinated by the positive atmosphere one seemed to find there. When the church needed help raising funds for its new complex, I contacted pianist Giovanni, who eagerly agreed to put on a concert to raise funds. It was a beautiful night of music, and Giovanni told the crowd he was doing it because, "Mike Henle asked me to help, and I said I'd be happy to."

A couple of days after the concert, Deacon Mike asked me if I'd speak to the people of the church. He wanted me to relate to the people what I had gone through and just how thankful I was to have my health.

For the first time in my life, I had the opportunity to speak to a group of people without having to worry about falling on my face. It was a new thing for me, and I welcomed the opportunity. I quickly began putting together a speech that people would find interesting and informative.

I hadn't ever given any thought to giving a speech. But the more I thought about it, the more interesting I thought this story had become. It was a good story with a warm and wonderful ending, an inspirational journey where the good guy finally wins.

We agreed that I'd give the speech at 4 p.m. Mass on a Saturday.

I was selected along with another young girl who had undergone a life-changing experience.

Deacon Mike introduced me to about six hundred people, and I calmly walked to the podium of St. Joseph's.

I told the story of the many years of ill health, and tried not to dwell on the bad. I wanted badly for people to know that I considered myself the luckiest man on the face of the earth. I told the story of the seizure that drove me to the ground while we were completing the house. I spoke of the book in the library at the University of San Diego and the meeting the following morning with the little fella named Dr. Aung. I told how Dr. Aung encouraged me for the first time in my life that we could find the answer to the problem. I told the congregation how he and Dr. Thomas Waltz, along with the staff of Scripps Hospital, turned my life around.

"If you've got your health, please never take it for granted," I told the audience. "If you've got your health, everything else will fall into place. Take it from me when I tell you that there is absolutely nothing more important than your health. It's an unbelievable feeling when a sick man finally realizes what it's like to feel good for the first time in his life."

The audience seemed to be paying attention. You could hear a pin drop during the speech, which took about 30 minutes. I thanked the audience for their time, and returned to my seat, where several people patted me on the back. It felt good to inspire others.

We concluded the service, and I began walking out of the church. The response to the speech was incredible. I had apparently done my job.

Then, one woman walked up to me, extending her hand. "Mike, I just wanted to congratulate you on your speech," she said. "Also, I wanted to ask you about the doctor. Was that Andy Aung?"

I responded that indeed, it was Andy Aung who had helped me.

"Well, would you believe that we are cousins?" she said. "We grew up together."

I couldn't believe it. Talk about a small world. Then, the woman told me a fascinating story about her cousin and my friend, Andy

Aung.

"You know, Andy used to be a heart doctor," she continued. "Then, he discovered that so many Orientals were having seizures. Because of that, he switched from being a heart doctor to a neurologist."

Praise God, I thought to myself.

CHAPTER 28
WORD OF MY RECOVERY
BEGINS TO SPREAD

As the healing period continued, my business continued to prosper. And as word traveled that I had apparently been cured of my long bout with epilepsy, the phone began to ring from others who needed help.

One call came from Clark County Commissioner Jay Bingham, whose friend, Robert Eliason, had been beaten badly by a burglar. The beating delivered with the handle of a flashlight, left Eliason, a father of four, with bad seizures.

Prior to the burglary at his home in North Las Vegas, Eliason had been healthy. Out of nowhere came the beating to be followed by the awful seizures.

Once I had made contact with Eliason, I called Scripps for help. As usual, the people there were sympathetic and eager to help. They had to know me almost on a first-name basis by now.

Eliason and his wife Peggy arrived at the house. We had never met before and became instant friends. We flew to San Diego, and journeyed up the coast to Scripps.

The next day, I led the young couple into the hospital, where we found our way to Dr. Aung's office. As luck would have it, Dr. Aung and I would cross paths in the hallway. He asked how I was doing, and I told him just fine. I explained that I had brought a friend to him for help.

A short time later, Eliason began suffering another seizure only minutes before his appointment with Aung. Eliason would later discover the value of Dr. Aung and the charm of Scripps Hospital, where nurses told him they'd simply send him the bill.

Eliason began getting his life back together, thanks to Dr. Aung and the people of Scripps.

And one day while at a conference, my beeper went off. A man named David Cox, a prominent Las Vegas man, called because his wife was having terrible problems with seizures. She was having reactions to Dilantin and was frightened of the fact that brain surgery was a possibility in her life. I assured David Cox that I'd stop by his house later in the afternoon. His wife was shaken badly. Did I ever know what she felt like. They must have been married for at least 40 years, and this was the first time the couple had faced such adversity.

"The only time I've been in the hospital is to have my children," Mrs. Cox would say. "I'm very scared."

I would later discover that three members of the church I attended were also suffering from seizures. And five years later, epilepsy would reach the headlines when U.S. Olympic track star Florence "Flo-Jo" Joyner would die of a grand-mal seizure while in her sleep.

My first grand-mal seizure also came while I was asleep. In Flo-Jo's case, she suffocated from the seizure. My family shuddered when the news hit the airwaves.

I'd also learn that two members of our parish were to have brain surgery. Charlene Sawyer was headed for UCLA for brain surgery, after being misdiagnosed for several years with multiple sclerosis. When Charlene related to me that doctors had previously thought she had MS, I explained that one had also suggested that my problem had been the same dreaded disease. Her brain tumor, apparently lying undiagnosed for many years, was removed and she would later recover to a wonderful life free of anguish and worry.

Another young woman named Krista Richardson was facing brain surgery because of a seizure disorder. The mother of two young children, she had been badly hampered by seizures for quite some time.

Finally, long-time friend Bobbi Grippo was rushed to University

Medical Center, after suffering a grand-mal seizure. Doctors removed a brain tumor and she, too, seems to be doing fine now.

When Deacon Mike Heidenreich asked me if I'd speak with Krista about her surgery, I eagerly told him I'd do anything I could.

I saw Krista at church, and offered my hand. I told her that I knew exactly what she was going through since I had been there. I also told her that I, too, had been scared before the surgery, but the end result was that I was seizure-free. Krista seemed to appreciate the chance to speak with someone who had gone through the same procedure that she was facing. She was headed for Arizona for the surgery, and I told her that I'd pray for her.

A short time later, Charlene and Krista had their surgeries. Both recovered nicely. Charlene no longer had to live with the constant fear that she had MS and Krista's seizures subsided, as she turned her attention to her family.

I finally began to discover that I hadn't been alone in my battle with epilepsy. Several people called for help and each time I attempted to let them know that I knew exactly what they were going through. In each instance, I remembered Sue Mortal, who counseled me after having her brain surgery at UCLA.

A very busy PR person, I could easily have been the "flack" for Scripps. Before long, I had sent several people to see Dr. Aung, including my wife's cousin, who could not find help in Las Vegas.

In each case, people came back to Las Vegas thankful for the opportunity to meet with Andy Aung. In each case, people came home refreshed and with a new spirit in their life.

My journey was continuing, and helping provide some sort of guidance to others who were experiencing epilepsy proved to be very satisfying.

CHAPTER 29
MARK NOVEMBER 10, 1997
ON THE CALENDAR

It has always baffled me why people will take drugs when they do not have to. Those who seem to want to ruin their lives with cocaine, marijuana or alcohol absolutely amaze me.

So, it was on Nov. 10, 1997 that I marked another day on the calendar in my continued recovery. Almost three years since the surgery, I would raise my arms in victory as sweet as anything I had ever celebrated. It was like a marathon runner crossing the line after more than twenty-six miles of grueling pain. It was on that day that a call from Scripps Hospital gave me the green light to end the prescription drugs I had been taking since I was fifteen years old. For thirty-one years, I had been taking one drug or another and none of them seemed to work.

The final recovery had taken longer than expected, because I had quit taking the phenobarbital before the two-year span after the surgery. I suddenly went into withdrawals and everyone noticed that something was wrong. Kate Culliton had warned me that it would take two years to get off the phenobarbital.

As I walked into Scripps for my check-up, I ran into her. When I told her that I thought I had goofed by going off the phenobarbital, she immediately cringed. "Don't tell me you went off your meds already," she said, adding that such a move could have serious consequences.

A short time later, I'd meet with Dr. Aung, who informed me that I was very fortunate that I did not have a seizure. I had to begin taking the drug again, again weaning myself off a little at a time.

To borrow a line from Frank Sinatra, I had tried to do it "my way." I almost learned the hard way that "my way" wasn't the best way.

The bottom line was that I was cured fully this time. The call from Scripps solidified that.

"Mike, didn't we do a right-side lobectomy on you?" asked Jeff Horst, who worked with Kate in Neurology at Scripps. Together, Jeff and Kate had been absolute lifesavers in our efforts to turn my life around.

"Yeah, that's it," I responded, not knowing what I was about to hear.

"You haven't had any problems, have you?" Jeff asked.

"Oh, it took me more than two years before I honestly started feeling human, but other than that, I'm fine," I said.

"Well, that's wonderful," Jeff said. "Dr. Waltz performed the same surgery on a man not long ago, and he suffered a blood clot. Dr. Waltz had to operate again to remove the clot, and now the patient is having trouble. He doesn't know the difference between day and night, and he can't sleep."

Once again, I thanked the Good Lord. I had problems, but nothing like this. I had lived in total fear upon returning home, because of the possibility that something might go wrong after being released from Scripps.

"Dad, it's a good thing they never told you something like this could happen," said our twenty-two-year-old son John. "You would never have had the surgery."

Never could anything have been truer. I had no way of knowing who the patient was, but felt as though he was my best friend. There could be no greater nightmare than having to go through brain surgery again.

But the bottom line was that I was fine, and for the first time in thirty-one years, I began to feel what it was like to be without drugs.

An incredible sense of inner peace had slowly become a part of my life. I wanted to travel to the highest mountain and scream to the world. The shackles had been removed, and I truly felt as though I had received my greatest boost.

On the day before Thanksgiving, I had great reason to be thankful. No more drugs, with the slight exception of an occasional over-the-counter pill to sleep.

I was no longer a prisoner of the prescription drug business. Perhaps it was only important to me, but what a victory. I felt as though we had just conquered another huge enemy.

One by one, little by little, the recovery had continued. The handcuffs were being released again and I could live a normal life. Suddenly, I could see the big picture and enjoy life.

The sounds of birds chirping seemed crisper and the beauty of the mountains literally jumped out at me. I had missed that sort of thing, and never really had the chance to experience life.

I was free now. I could live and I could cherish life.

I remember back in the 1960s hearing the late New York Yankee great Lou Gehrig say that he considered himself the luckiest man on earth, even though he was dying at the time.

I was no longer dying a slow death, but living a strong new life. The terror had been removed from my life and I was officially walking out of this jail cell called epilepsy.

For a man who made his living behind the keyboard, there was no word strong enough to describe the feeling of good health.

The trees were greener and the sky was bluer. The sermons at church were making more sense and my family was more important than ever before.

I'd sit and shed a tear, but it wasn't a tear of sadness. It was a tear of happiness.

To borrow a word from my kids, it was nothing less than "awesome."

CHAPTER 30
JUST WHAT THE DOCTOR DIDN'T ORDER

On December 19, 1998, I had decided to head for Las Vegas Motor Speedway, where I was employed as Media Relations Director. One of the "spiffs" related to the track was the chance to participate in auto racing.

And on this day, I had been invited to run a Legends racecar owned by Bobby Ruppert on the LVMS 3/8-mile paved track in the northeast valley near Nellis Air Force Base. Life was going good and I was free of any complications whatsoever of the woes that had plagued more for more than thirty-five years.

It was a cold and windy day, with a wind chill that made the day feel much colder than it actually was. When the wind combines with the cold in Las Vegas, the chill literally runs right through you.

Despite the bad weather, I thought I'd head for the track and take Ruppert up on his invitation. About halfway there, I suddenly felt ill. My arms hurt and so did my neck and back. My throat was raw and I just felt lousy. It happened so suddenly. Surely, I thought, I was catching the flu. Later that evening we were to have our annual Christmas party at the house. My day and night were to be ruined by a bug that generally seemed to reach its peak during the Christmas holidays.

I've always enjoyed fiddling with racecars, although I've certainly never displayed any talent behind the wheel. In fact, if the scars I have aren't because of surgery, they are the result of rolling nearly everything I've touched from go-karts to desert "quads."

With the chills running all through my body and the aches getting worse by the minute, I was in a quandary. Las Vegas—a twenty-four-hour city with as many twenty-four-hour emergency rooms as it has 7-11 convenience stores—had doctors' offices all over town.

My first inclination was to stop into a "Quick Care" and see a doctor. I'd get a shot, a prescription for some pills and get myself back on track. Then, I'd head for the track for some fun.

But for every emergency room that I passed, I kept thinking that I was nearing the time that I was to meet Ruppert at the track. I figured the best thing to do was scurry to the track, get my "fix"of auto racing and finally head for the doctor's office.

I had not been sick for too long, and the timing couldn't have been worse. With a busy schedule facing me, the last thing I needed was a case of the flu.

I arrived at the track, only minutes before Ruppert. The wind was worse and the temperatures had dipped even further. The wind chill had to be in the thirties and I cringed at the idea that I'd accept a ride in a racecar. At seventy mph and no windshield, I was sure to make this illness even worse.

I was certain my fever had climbed to about one hundred and one degrees. While the winds were cold, my body felt like it was burning up. It was classic influenza, and I just knew that I'd have to call someone to come take me home.

Ruppert showed up, asking me if I was ready to climb into the racecar. I didn't share with him the fact that I was sick and simply accepted the driver's suit.

My God, you're out of your mind, I told myself. *By the time everyone starts showing up at the house tonight, you'll be the life of the party. You'll be in bed, while everyone else is having a great time.*

I'd be the worst host in history. I could just hear it now. Everybody in town would be giving me the devil.

Ruppert opened the door, and I climbed inside the tiny car. I started the engine and guided myself toward the track. When the track official gave me the go-ahead, I proceeded onto the track in Ruppert's little powerplant.

As I accelerated, I noticed that my legs were killing me. I headed down the straightaway and started to pick up RPMs. As I headed into the turns, I noticed that driving a Legends Car was tantamount to running a go-kart, except that it had more power.

And in my case, the Legend car had a roll bar. That was a big "must" when I was behind the wheel of most anything.

I spun the car twice in ten laps and was waved off the track. Ruppert wiped his brow and thanked me for not crashing his No. 47 Legends Car.

I climbed out of the car, thankful that I hadn't made contact with the wall. I took the helmet off and the darnedest thing struck me. As dumb as it sounded, the fever was gone and so were the aches and pains. I unzipped the driver's suit and sat there in amazement. I was honestly afraid to say anything about the fact that my illness was gone. I felt just fine, although the weather was still cold and windy.

It finally hit me. The flu bug that had dominated me one hour earlier was literally gone. I couldn't believe it, and wasn't about to say anything. People would think that I had lost my marbles. Those who knew that I had endured brain surgery—and Ruppert was one of them—would think one of the wires had come loose again in my skull.

The next day, I called track physician Dr. Dale Carrison. I figured that I could tell him how the flu bug had disappeared after riding in a racecar and that he wouldn't laugh me out of town. While I was afraid to tell people of my experience, I felt comfortable talking with Dr. Dale.

"You may be on to something," said Dr. Dale, who was an FBI agent before a "mid-life" crisis led him to medical school. "That may have been the adrenaline rush."

It made all the sense in the world. The movie *Patch Adams* with Robin Williams specifically dealt with laughter and fun times as cures for illness, although the medical society didn't agree with the philosophy. Stress has played a part in so many illnesses, including cancer.

Laughter and good times were free. Nobody needs a trip to the pharmacist for that cure. You just need to be around happy and positive people. And for the life of me, Dr. Dale Carrison was the only doctor I knew who smiled often. He had fun with life—and I had never seen him sick.

In fact, I once referred to him as the "Patch Adams of auto racing" in a feature story I wrote about him. His theory about life was so well accepted that he was named the "Nevada Physician of the Year" in 1997.

I had been so accustomed to heading for the traditional doctor's office when I started feeling badly, even though the end result had generally been that I didn't feel any better two days later. I was amazed that I had accidentally discovered the cure for my illness.

I hadn't really been sick this time. I was stressed and while most doctors would never prescribe fun and laughter as medication, it had done the trick for me. I had again "tripped" across the answer to a medical problem on my own.

I often gave speeches for the track about the fun people had at the track. A short time later, I was to attend a Lion's Club luncheon at Canyon Gate, a country club in the southwest portion of the Las Vegas valley. On my way to the function, I called the people of the Richard Petty Driving Experience and asked for a complimentary one hundred and seventy-mile ride in a racecar as a door prize.

Walking up the steps to Canyon Gate, a thought suddenly struck me. Las Vegas, a town where people run full speed from the time they get up until the time they go to bed, was the stress capital of the world—and I had the ticket for the cure.

I gave a short speech about the track and told the gathering that we were about to draw a raffle ticket for a ride in a Richard Petty racecar. When I drew the winner's name, I held up the ticket and congratulated the man.

"You have bad days, don't you?" I asked, drawing a "What in the hell are you talking about?" look.

"Yeah, of course," was the response.

"Then, I want to you to take this certificate for a ride in a Richard Petty ride and remember one thing," I said. "Do not use it in the event of a good day. Save it for the day when the boss is yelling at you or the checkbook is upside-down. When you can't take anymore abuse, grab the certificate and head for the Richard Petty Driving Experience. I promise you that it will turn your bad day into a good one."

The guy looked at me with a dumbfounded look. I then explained my own personal story of riding in Ruppert's racecar and how I had immediately recovered from "influenza" only a few weeks earlier. When I told the crowd the story, it all made sense.

"Just consider this your prescription to good health," I said, "Call me Dr. Henle."

The crowd had no idea that I had spent so many years sick and that it took an absolute miracle to save me. That was my own little secret.

A couple of months later when I was having my own bad day, I headed for the infield and climbed into a Richard Petty racecar to get the cobwebs out of my head. I never gave a thought to going to a doctor's office.

Long-time Las Vegan Mel Larson took me about one hundred and seventy mph for four laps and I climbed out of the car feeling just fine. I had forgotten what was bothering me when I arrived for the ride. It worked like a charm and there was no fear of side effects from medication.

Oh, I could get hooked on this medication, but this time, that was fine.

I was having the time of my life more than five years after life changing surgery. Life was good.

Dear God, it was good to be alive—and healthy at the same time.

CHAPTER 31
IT IS INDEED A SMALL WORLD

Some thirty-seven years earlier at the age of thirteen, I had donated a small amount of money to a multiple sclerosis telethon that featured veteran boxer Archie Moore. During the telethon in Northern California, Moore read a poem that he had written about Cassius Clay.

A few days later, an envelope arrived in the mail complete with a card thanking me for my donation and the handwritten poem Moore had composed about Clay during the telethon. The envelope and its contents followed me from one place to another. I had lost many things, but the Archie Moore memorabilia was something that I just happened to hold on to. Through my many years of moving around, that envelope from the legendary prizefighter remained with me.

While attending the fights in June of 2000 at the Hard Rock Hotel and Casino, a woman sat down next to me and we started talking. As luck would have it, the woman was J'Marie Moore, daughter of Archie Moore, and a professional boxer. I immediately started telling J'Marie about the poem her dad had sent me nearly four decades earlier.

"You won't believe this," I told J'Marie. "But I have a poem that your dad wrote clear back in 1963 that he sent me after a telethon in Sacramento. Did you know that he was quite a poet?"

J'Marie assured me that she knew her dad was a poem writer. When we further discussed the idea, we both became fascinated at how this had all found its way to a boxing arena in Las Vegas. J'Marie said she'd call me sometime and we'd talk about her dad and the envelope he had sent me.

About three weeks after seeing J'Marie, the call came. In an even more ironic set of circumstances, I discovered that J'Marie had gone to college at the University of San Diego—where I had found the book that led to my recovery from epilepsy. The Moores lived in San Diego, not far from Scripps, and the family still owned the home. In fact, J'Marie said her dad's boxing ring was still in the backyard.

J'Marie then informed me her dad had died in 1998. My mouth literally hit the floor when she said her dad had been suffering from mini strokes—and he died of a grand-mal seizure. I could not believe my ears.

Seizures had indeed become a bigger problem than I had ever imagined —for many others. I was free of the worries and the mysteries of the disorder. Every day I thought about how lucky I was at least two or three times.

In fact, during the writing of this manuscript, I usually kept the contents with me during my day's travels. If the day went upside down or there were simply too many people screaming about one thing or another, I found that I could stop what I was doing, go to any chapter in the manuscript and relax. It just put everything in perspective for me, no matter what had driven me to the book.

Reading any part of the manuscript helped me realize what was important in life. I had survived a wicked ordeal and finally realized that it was time to be proud of myself. People had died from the disorder, but I was living a full life.

I suddenly discovered that more and more people wanted to hear the story of my battle with and eventual victory over epilepsy. One Las Vegas television station interviewed me during a half-hour show and CBS radio conducted another interview that aired on Sunday mornings over a couple of its stations.

In every case, people were fascinated in the battle and the eventual waving of the checkered flag. I suddenly started to realize that this was indeed a very good story—and my telling of it seemed to help others. I have always been someone who loved helping people. People seemed to find an inspiration in my unwillingness to give up—and I thought back about the conversation I had with Sue

Mortal, who had brain surgery at UCLA to end her life of seizures. She had been my inspiration and now I could be the same to others.

One day, I dropped by to see a long-time friend named Ron Ragona, thinking that I'd leave a copy of the manuscript off for him and his wife, Cheech.

I happened to run into Cheech some time later—and her response to the manuscript brought a whole new light to the story.

"Mike, I loved your book," Cheech said, giving me a hug. "And I have to tell you that it helped me in my battle with cancer."

I had no idea that Cheech had been ill—and the fact that my story helped her really opened my eyes. It brought back memories of the days when I was a writer for the *Las Vegas Review-Journal*. When people said a story I had written either helped them or brought sunshine to their day, I knew my job had been done correctly. There's simply no explanation for the satisfaction gained out of helping others through the written or spoken word.

My life continued to sail along pretty well, as I gained more confidence that the epilepsy was indeed a part of my life that was over with. Without the worry of seizures gripping my every move, I noticed that my confidence had gotten better.

I didn't panic about things like I had in the past, even when getting blind-sided by an unexpected event in my life. I told friends that recovering from the disorder and the surgery was hard and I had survived it—and everything else almost seemed insignificant.

Said one friend, "Just remember that which does not kill you will make you stronger."

My goodness, I thought. If that's the case, I must be very strong now.

I had grown to understand that I needed to relax more than before and I longed for views of the ocean. Kate Culliton, my clinician at Scripps, told me in 2000 that I really didn't need to come back for more tests, but was always welcomed if I just wanted to see some friends. I always remembered that, almost looking at Scripps and the ocean as my safety blanket should there come a time when I needed to regroup and relax.

In the meantime, I had referred enough people to Dr. Aung and Scripps that I joked to some that I was going to start my own shuttle service to the Southern California medical facility. But each time people came back telling me of their experiences at Scripps, I breathed another sigh of relief and felt good about my good deed.

There had been a huge weight lifted from my shoulders, something I didn't even know I had shouldered when I was sick. And with that weight taken off my shoulders and out of my mind, there was a chance to enjoy life —and help others at the same time.

CHAPTER 32
A DIFFERENT KIND OF WAR

For several weeks, I had known that I needed a vacation. I kept telling Carmen that I needed to go to the beach for a while, relax and gather my senses. The ocean had always been good to me; soothing my nerves and helping me make sense of things.

I called Kate Culliton at Scripps, and told her I would like to come down to stop by and see her and everyone else at the hospital. I always knew that going to Scripps would help me kind of count my blessings and regroup.

I went to someone at Saturn and requested a car to drive, loaded my golf clubs in the trunk and headed down the road. I took my cellular with me to stay in touch with home, but really needed to see another sun set in the ocean and hear the kind words of the folks at Scripps.

I grabbed another copy of the manuscript and headed down I-15. When I got to San Diego, I was greeted with a sign announcing that I was on Archie Moore Memorial Highway. I instantly thought about the poem he had written and sent to me so many years before—and the grand-mal seizure that had later taken his life.

When I got to San Diego, my first thought was to head for the wharf and get some seafood. However, I found myself journeying to Scripps right off the bat, if for nothing else to simply walk down the hallways and see smiling faces.

Perhaps it might seem strange to others, but I kind of felt like I was going home. In fact, it was a home. It was somewhere that had opened up its arms for me, just like my stepmom who had died on Memorial Day weekend of 2000.

It had been a rocky year, although my income had been good. Without warning, my stepmom died of a stroke the Friday before Memorial Day.

And until my dying day, I will never forget that it was my stepmom and my friends at Scripps who never wavered when I needed help. Neither of them knew much about me when we first met, but both offered a helping hand when I needed one.

I never referred to my stepmom as anyone other than "Mom." When my father and she married more than thirty years ago, she agreed to take me in, if I needed a home. And when I needed somewhere to go, Mom was waiting for me on the sidewalk with open arms even though she had never laid eyes on me before. She took one look at me, put her arms around me and said, "Welcome home."

The people of Scripps had done the same for me as Mom. When they found out I needed help in 1994, all they wanted to know was how long it would take to get to the clinic in LaJolla, California.

And when I got to Scripps, the doors opened up for me—and so did a new life.

With that in mind, I headed for Scripps on this hot July day. After I arrived at the clinic, I parked the car. I walked up the driveway and as I passed a part of the parking lot, something suddenly struck me. As I looked toward the ocean, I was reminded that the area where I was then walking was the precise spot where I had my last seizure on December 5, 1994. I slowed down for a few seconds and noticed that I had tears in my eyes. There were goose bumps on my arms, as I relived that day in my mind.

I remember stumbling, as I tried to fight off a strong seizure. I remember Carmen and the kids stopping to help me. And most of all, I remember Carmen telling me the demons were taking their last shots at me, because they would be eliminated from my life the next day. I will never forget that I honestly didn't think the seizures would ever end.

But most of all, I remember that seizure in the parking lot on December 5, 1994 would be the last seizure I'd ever have. The surgery I was about to experience would stop the epilepsy right in its tracks.

It was almost as though I was walking past a monument marking a historic battle or event. In a sense, it was a historic event, at least in my life. It was the last time that I had squared off against epilepsy, the last time that I ducked and weaved to avoid the punches of the disorder.

I continued my walk and headed down the hallway for the office of my neurosurgeon Dr. Thomas Waltz.

"Uh, excuse me," I said upon entering his office. "Is Sandra here?"

Sandra was Dr. Waltz's secretary and I had told her earlier that I'd be down.

"No, I'm sorry. Sandra is out ill today," was the response from the friendly receptionist.

"Is Kate here?" I asked.

There working away behind the computer was Kate Culliton, that big smile on her face. She didn't realize it was me, because I had shed my beard since the last time I had been to Scripps.

I had a copy of the manuscript for Dr. Waltz, and when I began to sign a note to him, Kate realized that one of her old patients had come to visit.

"You look twenty years younger," she said amazed. "I didn't even recognize you."

We all had a good chat, speaking of the surgery and the disorder we had all defeated together. Kate recalled that she was pregnant at the time of my surgery and I would later think to myself that two new people were brought into the world at about the same time—Kate's new baby and me with my newfound health.

Kate told me that she found it interesting that I actually had been kind of lost without my seizures when I first got out of Scripps December 13, 1994. I recalled the conversation and agreed that it was rather interesting. It sounded kind of strange, but I understood the analogy. I guess I just had to adjust to an entirely different lifestyle and everything about my life actually required adjustment.

I told her that I had related epilepsy to a war. While you're glad to get out of a long war, soldiers must have flashbacks at the same time. That's kind of how I related to the epilepsy. I hated the enemy, but admired its fight.

I had finally won, but not without a long battle. Good Lord, I even had battle scars, such as the one on the palm of my left hand the time I had grabbed a hot pan during a seizure. Then, there was the light scar on the right side of my head where the team at Scripps carefully opened my skull to remove the damaged temporal lobe that produced the seizures.

We discussed the surgery and the results of the procedure. We talked about the fact that the last seizure I had was the day before the surgery standing in front of Scripps. Kate recalled that I had an aura after the surgery, but never a full-blown seizure.

And it was then that I discovered that more than two hundred surgical procedures like the one I had had been performed. I was the only one that anyone knew of who did not have at least one seizure following the surgery.

Dr. Aung said the success rate of the surgery was sixty to sixty-five percent. He then told me my surgery had been a true success story. Later during my visit, I'd drop by to see Dr. Waltz to have a short consultation. Most important, though, was the fact that I needed to tell him thank you for all he had done. Until my most recent trip to Scripps, I had forgotten that the last time I had seen Dr. Waltz was before I left the hospital.

Some people had told me in the past that I was a medical miracle. After sitting in Dr. Waltz's office on that day, I again realized that I was indeed a very fortunate person. No other health problem could have ended as quickly as the one that almost ran my life into the ground.

After speaking with Kate for about ninety minutes, I decided to head for the beach. I found a place at Solana Beach north of Scripps and headed for the surf.

Just to sit and gather my thoughts, I placed myself on a rock and soaked up the sun and the sounds of the ocean. It was so soothing and watching the waves rolling in, I thought back of the years of being sick. The waves came in clusters—and so had the seizures a few years before. But while the waves come in clusters, you at least knew they were headed your way.

Seizures had come in waves, too, but there was never much of a warning. When they wanted to knock you down, you were at their mercy. Seizures were rude and unforgiving, choosing to embarrass you in front of friends or place you in danger while doing things like driving a car.

The ocean at least warned you it would knock you down. Epilepsy had no mercy when it was walking over my life.

While speaking on the cellular with Fran Minnozzi, a client from Las Vegas, I was confronted by a lifeguard. "Sir, you had better move," she warned. "This may be the dumbest thing you have ever done. Look at the signs."

I had not seen the sign that warned of a cliff that was about to collapse. I was sitting below it and didn't even know it. I was so busy enjoying the ocean I had just walked by the warning.

"Tell her you survived brain surgery, so something like a falling cliff is no big deal." Fran laughed.

In truth, she was right. I had dodged so many bullets in my life that I was indeed a medical miracle. About one year earlier, I rolled my four-wheeler about twenty miles from our home in Las Vegas and had no helmet to protect my skull. In spite of the bad rollover, I managed to right side the badly damaged four-wheeler with a little help from a guy who just happened to be riding through the middle of the desert in his Baja Bug, I rode the machine home.

When I walked in the door, my face and head were badly cut and my shoulder was hanging from the break. It wasn't long before I was in the emergency room.

"Well, I can see where you've had brain surgery," said the x-ray technician, pointing to a cut that would require several stitches to close the wound—right on top of where an indention in the skill was left from the surgery. About a week later, I needed surgery on my right shoulder to repair a badly broken collarbone.

All those times just seemed to slowly find their way through my mind, as I enjoyed the surf—in a safer location.

I remembered the good times we had with the kids, wonderful people of Scripps and the time I spent relaxing by the ocean.

As I watched the sun disappear into the ocean on this beautiful day, I crossed myself and thanked God for everything I had been given in life.

Chapter 33

A Story Worth Hearing

Nearly ten years later, I still marveled at what an absolute miracle this entire experience had been. After this long, I was convinced that everything was indeed okay and that I was fully seizure-free.

While I had been cautious in the past that I could have another seizure, I was indeed okay. I could write about the experience freely and I could encourage others, because I was indeed a survivor.

There are no more questions to ask anymore. No more prescription drugs were needed anymore and I could maintain my pace without worrying about a seizure knocking me on my backside.

All I needed to do was check in with the people of Scripps one or two times a year just to say hello.

While visiting Scripps again, I had the opportunity to meet with everyone involved in changing my life. I just felt it was necessary to say thanks once in awhile.

It had been my feeling that we just don't show our gratitude enough anymore. I wanted to be certain that I didn't fall into that same trap.

What I have always loved about Scripps is that they've never been too busy for me. Whether it's a phone call or a visit, there's always been time to exchange pleasantries.

I always felt it is important to just stop by and say hello. In my heart, I have always believed that my good friends at Scripps are as happy as I am that things turned out so well, so I try to make certain that they know they're in my thoughts and prayers.

"My gosh. How long has it been since we operated on you?" asked Dr. Waltz, whose pleasant smile has always been wonderful to see. He seemed as delighted as I that we could look back with such fond results of a very serious surgery.

"I thank my lucky stars every day of my life," I said to Dr. Waltz. We talked for about thirty minutes and discussed the surgery. Although it may sound a little strange, I have always wished that I could have seen a film of the procedure. Since that wasn't possible, the next best thing was listening to the marvelous gentleman who performed the surgery.

Dr. Waltz explained that the surgery had also helped many, many people. The success of the procedure was excellent and most of those whose seizures didn't end completely at least experience decreased seizure activity.

Our visit included conversations with Kate Culliton, as well as Dr. Aung, both whom expressed their delight to see me again.

However, more than anything, I truly wanted to know how I had changed. We had all experienced this battle, this victory and this massive life-changing experience.

I needed help from those close to me, so I reached out to family and close friends.

MY FATHER'S BATTLES MADE ME A BETTER PERSON

BY JOHN HENLE

I look back on my relationship with my father and see two different periods of time. One is a time of uncertainty, strength, and strong will. The other is a time of confidence, new beginnings, and faith. It is amazing to look back and see how I learned how to cope with challenges in life by relating my challenges with my dad's battle with epilepsy.

Everyday there are challenges we deal with that cause stress. I have learned that no matter what the situation is, it is not a big deal, unless it involves my family. Work, school, or problems with day-to-

125

day things are not the same as dealing with epilepsy each and every day. My dad's battles showed his strength and strong will to support a family and enjoy the job that he did. Giving up was something that was never displayed to me or to my brothers. My dad might have felt that way inside, but he never displayed any regrets or feelings of discouragement to his sons.

Growing up with epilepsy was just a part of my father that never seemed strange or abnormal. It was all I knew of him and seizures were a thing that was OK. We had times of playing basketball in the front yard with the neighborhood kids and having to stop because my dad would have a seizure. My friends would ask, "What is wrong with your dad?"

I never thought anything was wrong; it was just a part of him that had always been there.

When I got older I began to put myself in his shoes. I don't think I would have had the strong will that my father had. To wake up every morning and not know whether this is going to be the day that you had zero seizures or three seizures before dinner would be a heavy burden on my shoulders. I admire my father for being as strong as he was during this time. His strength and ability to bounce over each of the hurdles has guided me in my family life and professional career.

The second part of my relationship with my father was one that had a scary start. I almost missed the surgery because I had fall semester finals the next couple of days following his surgery. I did not decide to go to San Diego until the last moment. It did not hit me until it was almost too late that this was a very serious surgery and an inflection point in his life and mine.

The surgery went as planned and everything seemed to be OK. We returned to Las Vegas for the recovery period that lies ahead. My mother was the one who kept my father together. The same strong-will and never give up attitude was taking a toll on my father. This is the one time that my father had to take time to relax and rely on his family to keep things going. As my father says in his book, this was a time that was very challenging for himself and his family.

Seizures have not been a part of our family since that surgery at

Scripps. I thank those doctors who have made our lives better. This might sound strange, but seizures did make our family strong before the surgery. I might not have had the strength that I have now if I did not learn about the never give up attitude that my father has.

My father's new beginning has been refreshing to him and his family. There is a confidence that is now displayed due to the absence of seizures in his life. During this entire experience I have learned to never give up because you never know what could happen to change your life for the better. I do hope that this book helps others realize that they do have a chance because their faith and the help of others can make a difference. It has for me and it will for my children and my grandchildren.

MY DAD

BY JOE HENLE

Thinking of my father's life before his life saving surgery I am reminded of one of my favorite movies of all time, *Rocky IV*. His bout with epilepsy was much the same as the final scene in that great American movie. My dad, much like Rocky, turned out triumphant in the final round of his struggle with his debilitating disorder.

Growing up in Northern California, my father was subjected to a childhood where he was thrown into the realm of the "real world" much before the average child. In the early rounds of his life he was faced with a challenge to live with a volley of blows that definitely staggered him. At an early age he suffered from encephalitis. These early punches were the catalyst that set the stage for the next forty years, or in boxing terms, twelve rounds. However, just as in *Rocky IV*, he was able to strike back at his imposing menace by living the life of a normal child by succeeding in school, sports and developing a natural talent of writing.

Next came the middle rounds of his bout with epilepsy. It was here when he learned that plain guts and determination is the only thing that can get you through the toughest of times. During his mid-teen years he suffered a series of knockdowns that could have put him down for the ten count. With an alcoholic mother and a father who just could not take it anymore, he found himself alone. Eventually, he made it to Las Vegas, and through the middle rounds, a few points behind. This was all in the midst of cheap shots that should have compelled a referee of life to deduct points from epilepsy.

Then about the tenth and eleventh rounds my father and mother met each other and my two brothers and I were the byproduct of that loving relationship. During these rounds my dad realized that he had to hang on and take the punishing blows for the good of his family. Prescription drugs often softened these blows, but again it was his determination that allowed him to succeed. These rounds lasted nineteen long years until December of 1994 when he went in for surgery.

The twelfth round is the one that I remember best. It was definitely the shortest round of the battle but it climaxed in a way that not even Rocky and Ivan Drago could have matched. The morning of his surgery, I remember he had a series of seizures. My mother, like all good corner people do, gave my dad one of the best motivating statements I have ever heard. I cannot remember exactly what she said, but it was along the lines of, "They (seizures) are taking their last shots."

It was as if the disorder knew that it was on the verge of getting knocked out and it needed to give its all. But the disorder's efforts were in vain, as my dad went in and came out a winner with a vicious combination of guts and determination that left his arch enemy laying on the canvas defeated.

Because of his knockout victory, he can live the life free from a demon that often cheap-shotted below the belt or after the bell. Since that day I have noticed an aura of confidence emitting from his persona. But still his determination and good old fashion guts are the driving force in his life. Just remember when you think you are down and out, look at my dad and maybe you can realize that you, too, can succeed.

Carmen, my wife of thirty-two years, added this:

Before your surgery, you had a hard time with things mechanically. That has changed and you can read directions and put things together better than before. In addition, you have more confidence and more patience. Being able to finish your book is an example of your confidence. You don't get upset as easily as you used to and you go with the flow more now. As an example, when our house burned down in January of 2002, you were able to handle everything without freaking out. The fact that you were able to sell the home as-is shows your confidence. You're not the worrier that you were before.

My dad, Rudy, said I became an all-together different person after the surgery.

"I was really worried when you called and said you were having the surgery," he said. "It's a pretty critical operation. When somebody messes with your brain, that's very serious. Once you got past the critical stage, the changes have been amazing. Upon your transformation you have never been so good. Before you were always kind of fuzzy, whereas today you're bright. Everything seems to be okay. You're much more confident now. I was really worried when you were going to have another seizure, particularly when you were driving."

From my old sports editor Tom Dye came the following:

I have known Mike for thirty years and worked with him for nearly twenty. Before Mike had his operation, we used to call him "Mad Dog" because he was volatile and unpredictable. His friends worried about him because his condition caused him to black out. A new Mike emerged after his operation. He still has his trademark enthusiasm and energy and willingness to champion a cause, but he is more at peace and able to deal with life's problems. I've changed his nickname to "Mellow Dog."

Monica Caruso is a former co-worker of mine at the *Las Vegas Review-Journal* who worked across from me. She edited my copy and probably could see perhaps better than any one that I was really struggling. She offered the following:

As a friend and associate of Mike Henle for more than twenty years, I watched him grapple with the misery of undiagnosed and misdiagnosed illness. Mike's life was consumed with ongoing doctors' appointments and trips to the pharmacy to pick up prescriptions that never helped, while trying to maintain the semblance of a normal life devoted to his work in journalism and public relations, his beloved wife and sons, and his passion for motor sports. Because of his lengthy illness, and with no hope for relief, he was often frustrated, overwhelmed, unfocused and angry. His friends affectionately dubbed him "Mad Dog" because of his bouts of erratic, effusive behavior, but Mike was no madman.

At the persistent urging of his devoted family and friends, coupled with his own tenacity to find an answer, Mike finally got to bottom of his health problems and took courageous, bold action: brain surgery.

Since his successful surgery, Mike is a new man, cheerful and optimistic, yet humbled by the good fortune of regaining his health against the odds. He offers encouragement to the sick and depressed with stories of his own triumph. He is centered and focused, a better friend and family man for his experience. He has a story worth hearing.

EPILOGUE

There are two episodes in my life that I swore I would complete.

First, I was bound and determined that I would find the answer to my health problems. It took me getting knocked to the ground more times than I care to remember, but I didn't give up.

And finally, I made a commitment to myself in July 1995 that I would write a book about my experience. On a warm summer night, I walked into my office at home and started writing. I really had no idea where I was going, but I knew that I needed to finish the story.

When I mentioned the idea to a doctor at Scripps Hospital, he said the focus of the story was actually too narrow. I felt that finishing the book was important, if for no other reason than to give a copy to my family and my friends. While I may have trouble conveying my thoughts verbally, I've always been able to put them down on paper or in a computer.

My public relations company is called "The Idea Co." I've failed to finish projects enough times to need "The Follow Up Company" and this was one time when I wanted to complete the task.

When I completed the forward, I sent it to *Las Vegas Review-Journal* columnist John L. Smith, who like me, came to the *R-J* after working as a sportswriter at the *Las Vegas Sun*. I have always felt that John is the best columnist in Las Vegas history, and probably one of the finest writers in the country.

He writes with heart. Not many writers have that talent.

When John wrote the book *Running Scared....The Life and Treacherous Times of Las Vegas Casino King Steve Wynn*, I went to see him in October of 1995 at a book signing. I purchased the book and asked John if he'd sign it for me.

131

John wrote a wonderful note for me. He ended the greeting with a request that would honestly be the biggest encouragement I could receive to finish this book:

One of my favorite trivia questions. Who gave me encouragement when no one else would?
Mike Henle. Thank you for your friendship and support.

And then John would end the greeting that I would look at ten thousand times while attempting to finish *Through the Darkness: One Man's Fight to Defeat Epilepsy.*

John wrote, *Please finish your book.*

Every time I tired of writing the book and thought about throwing the whole thing in the trash, I looked at John's note. I'd reach for John's book, open the cover and his four words literally inspired me to keep going. It was that simple.

Coming from a journalist as talented as John L. Smith, those words meant a lot to me. Every writer in the country needs one reason to keep going and that literally drove me to complete it. If John L. Smith thought my story was a good one, that was good enough for me.

The truth is that I wanted to write the book for several reasons. First, it was a part of my life that needed to be completed. After so many years of struggling and finally finding a cure to my health problems, I felt it needed to be told. Finishing the book adds a sense of closure to a lifelong illness that was corrected only by a group of absolute miracle workers.

It proves that the good guy wins in the end. My team—my wife and three sons at my side, didn't give up during the war. We held together. During 1994, our plate was overflowing, apparently so we could be tested. We survived some very challenging times from the time we arose in the morning until the time we went to bed at night. Every day was an adventure, filled with the unknown.

Also, I felt my recovery was proof that people cannot give up. There is a reward at the end of a long fight, and I'm proof of that.

There could not be a more grateful or happy person than Michael Anton Henle, who is nothing more than a forty-eight-year-old man who has been working since he started selling newspapers on the streets of Carmel, California, at the age of seven.

Ironically, it was the age of seven when I had my first noticeable seizure. Perhaps I survived all those years because I kept my mind off the illness by working. Work has always been my greatest therapy.

But the truth is that finishing this book was the hardest task of my life. I first wrote the book, only to let it sit for quite some time. I pulled it out of the drawer one day and literally re-wrote the whole thing. It helped me during my recovery from brain surgery, because it allowed me to pour my feelings out—even if it was into a computer.

This story is not filled with medical language because I'm a simple person who had a simple goal. Hopefully, people can identify with the story and find reason to keep going. I've always gotten a lot more out of helping others than I have for receiving a paycheck. The problem with society today is that we're too busy to help one another, and that's very sad.

Had it not been for the people like Lynn and Art Dufresne, my parents, my wife and children and the people of Scripps, Lord only knows where I would be today. I was a wayward kid in more trouble than any of us knew, and a select group of people saw something in me.

People found time for me, and lent me their hands when I needed to be helped. We should all be so lucky.

Society has become overrun with greed nowadays. We are so busy chasing the dollar that we have forgotten to help our fellow man. We have failed to take time to thank people for what they do for us. The end result is that we have lost something, and the values of society are not what they used to be.

This book—no matter what is done with it—is intended to thank everyone for what they have done for me. I've been as guilty as anyone forgetting to offer a heartfelt sense of gratitude, so these writings are intended to let the world know how grateful I am for what I have.

This was written so that my family and my friends will have something that can be kept forever. It was written to remind us all that material belongings don't mean a thing if we don't have our health.

This isn't a simple thank-you card that will be thrown away after time. It's something that was written from the heart during all hours of the night. It was produced with the idea that it will hopefully inspire others to be thankful for what they have.

Reliving more than thirty-eight years of seizures was not easy. Reproducing that portion of my life by writing about it was very difficult. I trudged through the time, and writing about the seizures— especially the grand mals—was just awful. It brought back so many bad memories, including the fears suffered by my family and myself.

We couldn't go anywhere together without the fear of my having a seizure. We didn't talk about the problem until it arose, but we all undoubtedly shared the same concern. We constantly had a cloud over our heads, and we were never sure when the storm would hit.

It wasn't until I reached the portion of the book that told of my finding an answer to my illness while researching books at the University of San Diego Medical Library that I began to get moving. It was at that point that the words began to flow and I began to feel good about the book. I literally found new life and energy.

In a sense, I began to recover again at that point. I needed a strong faith to understand there was a reason for all of this. It was faith that kept me going before the surgery and after. Call it the Dale Carnegie outlook on life.

It was then that I used the CD from the motion picture soundtrack *Patch Adams* for the background music. Never in my life have I ever seen such a powerful movie and the music literally generated line after line out of me.

Rod Stewart's singing "Faith of the Heart" seemed to tell my own story, but I could identify with every song on the soundtrack. The whole movie is based on the belief that we need to take care of one another. A little understanding, a soft voice and a smile can combine for incredible healing powers.

In the end, it was the second breath I received from three people who reviewed portions of the book and added encouragement to finish the book.

Lynn and Art DuFresne, who lived across the street from me when I was a kid in Yuba City, Calif., now live in Oregon. When I e-mailed copies of some of the book, the response was always favorable.

It was Lynn and Art who guided me during some very difficult times when I was fifteen. When I had nowhere to go, they rescued me from an emergency room where I had gone to put my mother in the hospital. They gave me a roof over my head, and encouraged me to go live with my dad in Las Vegas.

My dad had remarried and the woman he wed literally saved both of our necks. Barbara Henle may have been my stepmother, but I have never referred to her as anything other than Mom. The first time she laid eyes on me, her first words were "Welcome home," something that I'd never forget.

Her being in Las Vegas for my dad literally led me to the beginning stages of an answer to my health problems. My dad and I had been through a lot, and her love and guidance were needed badly. She took both of us in and gave us reason to keep living.

My brother, Jim, (he's also my stepbrother, but we might as well be blood brothers) was the only other person to receive the book as it was being finished. His words of encouragement were also helpful. As soon as I heard from him, I'd start rewriting more chapters again—and again and again.

Jim and my mom died before the book had been published, but their importance in this victory was immeasurable.

It's very difficult for people to recognize their own story as being anything of any value. It took encouragement from many others, ranging from my family to the DuFresnes, to keep me going. If this book serves as inspiration in a very negative society, then the long hours included in it were worth it.

To borrow a few lines from "Faith of the Heart," it was a long road getting from there to here. It was a long time, but my time was finally near.

Nothing is in my way. They're not going to hold me down any more. I've got faith of the heart and I'm going where the heart takes me.

I have faith to believe I can do anything. No one is going to bend or break me.

I can do anything. I can reach any star. I have faith...faith of the heart. I've been through the darkness, but I finally have my day.

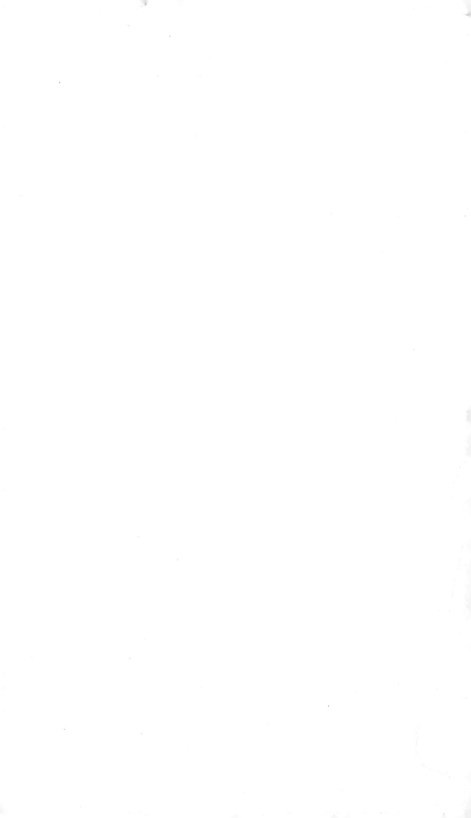

Printed in the United States
32971LVS00002B/43-123